SHIATZU

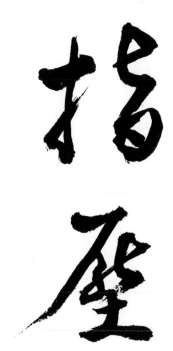

Japanese Finger Pressure for Energy, Sexual

J. B. LIPPINCOTT COMPANY • Philadelphia and New York

SHIATZU

by Yukiko Irwin
with James Wagenvoord

Foreword by M. Dorothea Kerr, M.D.
Illustrations by Raymond Burns

Vitality and Relief from Tension and Pain

U.S. Library of Congress Cataloging in Publication Data

Irwin, Yukiko.
   Shiatzu: Japanese finger pressure for energy, sexual
vitality and relief from tension and pain.

      1. Shiatzu.   I. Wagenvoord, James,
joint author.   II. Title.
RM723.S5I78   615'.822   75-17556
ISBN-0-397-01054-0
ISBN-0-397-01107-5 (pbk.)

*To the Memory of My Family
Who Became a Bridge
Between East and West*

As a practicing physician and psychiatrist, I have referred many patients for shiatzu therapy. I have found it an effective adjunct for tension disorders varying from pure emotional tension states to such ailments as shoulder and low back pain, migraine headaches and mild hypertension.

The sensations are difficult to describe but are similar to those experienced in mild hypnosis. One has a definite feeling of *working with* the body rather than *imposing on* the body as may occur with drugs and many technical procedures.

In treating all tension syndromes, one is looking for ways to help the patient relax, let down. I use many methods, including drugs, hypnosis, and exercise, as well as medical massage. Shiatzu, in my opinion, is a preferable type of medical massage as it induces a very deep relaxation with a gentle meeting of one's physical and mental states. As a treatment for today's tensions, an effective help like shiatzu is very welcome.

M. Dorothea Kerr, M.D.
Clinical Assistant Professor of Psychiatry
   Cornell University Medical College

Assistant Attending Psychiatrist
   Payne Whitney Clinic, New York Hospital

Foreword

Acknowledgments

I offer my deepest gratitude and admiration to Genevieve Young, without whom this book would not have been possible.

I am also indebted to Rebekah Harkness, who helped open a path for my practice in the West.

I am especially thankful to Aaron Frosch, who, as a friend, gave me wise legal counsel and assistance.

A special word of thanks goes to Martha Pate, Ph.D., who offered me her country place so that I could write in peace and quiet.

My warm appreciation goes to Kengo Minato, Jane Hsueh and Maimie Lee, who were a constant source of assistance, encouragement and friendship.

Contents

Part I

Shiatzu
to Maintain
Health
and
Vitality

Would you like to have more energy and vitality?

Would you like to feel more serene?

Would you like to free yourself from the pain of ailments such as headaches, lower back pain, constipation or tennis elbow?

Would you like to have more sexual vigor?

Would you like to look younger?

If your answer to each question is yes, and I cannot imagine anyone saying no, welcome to shiatzu. I believe that shiatzu should become an important part of your life. It can help you to relax, feel better, and increase your youthfulness and energy.

Shiatzu as a word is derived from the Japanese "shi" (finger) and "atzu" (pressure). As a health-keeping art, it is a product of 4,000 years of Oriental medicine, therapy and philosophy. It became the focus of my life when, as a young girl in Tokyo in the late 1940's, I first met a shiatzu therapist. He was an elderly man who had come to give my aunt treatment for debilitating headaches which had bothered her for months. After examining her, he determined that the professional and social pressures of her life had caused physiological and psychological tensions which produced and prolonged her pain. He claimed that by using shiatzu he could relax her tense muscles, eliminate her tension and bring a better flow of blood throughout her body. And after several months of intensive shiatzu therapy her headaches were gone and did not return. During this period I became extremely interested in the art of shiatzu, and the therapist encouraged me to learn from him. I was profoundly moved by his skill, sincerity and inner serenity and wanted to experience these things for myself. After studying with him, it was with his encouragement that I studied at the Nippon Shiatzu School for two

Chapter 1

Shiatzu: What It Is and Why It Works

years. After graduating, I received my accreditation from the Japanese Ministry of Health.

Since coming to the United States, I have tried to help people by working closely with several medical doctors in New York City. I have also served as the resident therapist with a major ballet company.

Now I offer you my thoughts and insights on basic shiatzu techniques so that you can learn the fundamentals and treat yourself and others. In the pages which follow I will show you how to maintain your health, receive shiatzu's exercise benefits, and treat simple, everyday aches and tensions.

But I must stress that this is a book for the layman—not a book for a person who wishes to learn and practice shiatzu professionally. Such a study involves more advanced technique and knowledge than any single book can offer. Work such as mine, as a professional, requires intensive training and is carried out under the supervision of medical doctors. The doctor diagnoses, and the professional therapist treats the patient in close consultation with the doctor.

Although shiatzu is widely known and practiced in Japan, it was virtually unknown in the West until acupuncture began receiving wide public attention. Acupuncture is the use of needles on key points (tsubas) of the body. The art of shiatzu is based upon the same body points, but instead of inserting needles it systematically applies pressure on these points by thumbs, fingers and palms. I often describe it by calling it acupressure. The best way to introduce you to this healing and life-enhancing art is to look briefly into its roots in ancient Oriental philosophy—the concept of Oneness.

Oneness means that the life of the universe and the life of an individual are essentially the same and are made from the same elements. According to the ancient Oriental philosophers, each life, everything in the universe, even the universe itself, follows the same life cycle. Yin and yang are the opposing forces of the universe which must be maintained in balance if Oneness is to be attained. Yin is a negative or minus force. Yang is positive. The moon is considered yin—the sun, yang. Night is yin—day is yang; water is yin—fire, yang. Within the concept of yin and yang there are no absolutes, and it is thought that although the forces are opposing they are also in harmony. For instance, man is yang to woman, yin. Since neither yin nor yang is an absolute, each contains the other, and everything is made of both yin and yang. Men and women both have male and female hormones.

It is also thought that yin and yang forces are not static; that they are changing constantly, and an excess of yin becomes yang and too much yang becomes yin. When water (yin) is frozen (yin), it becomes ice (yang).

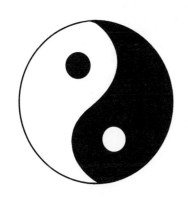

The symbol for yang and yin.

Since its beginnings, Oriental medicine has been closely related to the philosophy of Oneness and the idea of yin and yang forces of the environment and the body. The belief was that diminished health occurred only when the equilibrium between yin and yang was broken. The approach to healing was preventive, to keep the body in harmony. If, however, the harmony was lost, it had to be restored. This attitude of prevention has been carried down through the years to shiatzu, for it is first and foremost a method to maintain health and keep the body in harmony.

The ancient Chinese healers and philosophers made intensive studies of human ailments. The system which grew out of these studies was quite different from that developed by modern Western medicine thousands of years later. The Oriental approach is empirical: practices are based on experience and observation. The Chinese sages observed that certain ailments affected certain points on the surface of the body: various points became hot, cold, numb, hard, painful, oily, dry, discolored or stained. They located 657 such points on the body and observed that some of these points appeared to be related to one another. Acting like medical map makers, they charted the lines between these related points and determined that there are twelve pathways or meridians connecting the points on each half of the body. In addition to these twelve pairs of body meridians, they traced out two coordinating meridians which bisect the body. One, known as the meridian of conception, runs up from the base of the trunk, up the center of the abdomen, the center of the chest, and ends at a point in the front center of the lower jaw. The second, the governor meridian, begins in the center of the upper gum, traces up and over the center of the skull, down the spine, and ends at the base of the tailbone. The meridian of conception was so named because the sexual organs are located along this line. It acts mainly on yin energy. The governor meridian received its name because of the extreme significance of the spine as the main pillar of the body. It acts mainly on yang energy. These two bisecting meridians control the energy which flows constantly through the twelve pairs of body meridians. Interconnected, the twelve pairs of body meridians or pathways form the single energy system which maintains the health of the body.

The accuracy of the sages' observation is attested to by the fact that their idea of the functions of these meridians corresponds in many cases to the functions of the various networks discovered so many centuries later by Western medicine, i.e., the circulatory and nervous systems, the endocrine system, the reproductive system, etc.

The early sages believed that the meridians were pathways through which the energy of the universe circulated throughout the body organs and kept the universe and the body in harmony. They conceived that illness or pain occurred when the pathways became blocked, disrupting the energy flow and breaking the body's harmony. By inserting extremely fine needles into the body at the affected points on the pathways and into related points, they believed that the pathways' blockage was broken and the flow of energy was restored. They also believed that periodic treatment of a healthy person helped to preserve the flow of energy and to prevent illness. This grew into the science of acupuncture.

Over the years acupuncture has become a sophisticated medical discipline still based upon its early concept—that it is necessary to maintain balance between all areas of the body within itself as well as within the external environment.

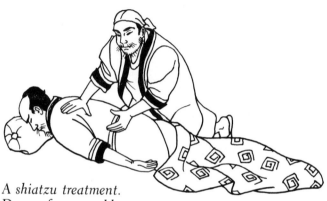

A *shiatzu treatment.*
Drawn from an old
Japanese woodcut.

Chinese acupuncture was introduced to Japan 1,300 years ago. Shiatzu developed during the eighteenth century in Japan as a combination of acupuncture and the traditional amma form of Oriental massage. Am (press) ma (stroke) was a simple pressing and rubbing of painful spots on the body by the fingers and palms of the hands. It was determined that instead of needles, direct thumb and finger pressure on the acupuncture meridian points would gain similar results. The points are, in effect, the floodgates which when stimulated with steady direct pressure keep the energy systems in motion. This innovation is regarded as the beginnings of shiatzu as we know it, although it was nearly two hundred years later, in the 1920's, that the name shiatzu became part of the Japanese language. Today there are over 20,000 licensed shiatzu therapists in Japan, and the art itself is a part of nearly every Japanese life.

Although shiatzu is closely allied to acupuncture and shares its effects on the body, I strongly favor shiatzu as an individual discipline for a normally healthy person. Acupuncture is primarily a way to treat ailments, while shiatzu's main function is to maintain health and well-being—although it does overcome many ailments and aches. Shiatzu is free of the risks of infection or rupture that are inherent in needle therapy. While it is not possible for a layman to give acupuncture, virtually anyone can learn the basic shiatzu techniques. And you can apply shiatzu to yourself easily.

There is one important warning, however, that you must keep in mind as you learn to give and receive shiatzu. Shiatzu should never be given to anyone who has a fever or infection, suffers from any kind of internal organ disorder, is susceptible to internal bleeding, for example from stomach or duodenal ulcers, or has a bone fracture.

Throughout this book I refer to the person receiving shiatzu, both self and partner, as "she" and "her." The reasoning is personal. Oriental medical charts and diagrams invariably are based upon a male form. The points are similar for both men and women and very simply I am tired of seeing references only to "he" or "him." Rather than clutter my descriptions with "either-or" I prefer to strike a blow, admittedly glancing and minor, for nonchauvinistic diagrams.

Whether you are a man or a woman, shiatzu can enhance your life. When it is used intelligently and consistently, in concert with proper diet and exercise, its purposes become its results. Muscles relax, pains are alleviated, nervous tensions diminish. Take advantage of it. You'll find that as an ancient sage once said, "Healthy thoughts and vitality spring from the healthy body."

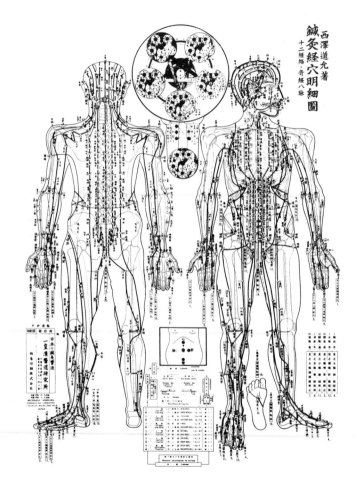

Illustration from a Japanese textbook on shiatzu, showing the points and meridians.

The fundamental philosophy of my work with shiatzu is giving, to ease another's pain, to make another person feel better.

We often take our hands and fingers for granted, but they serve us as a means of communication and a way to ease pain. When in love, people hold hands or touch each other. When one is in pain, one's hands reach directly to the area of the pain. Being at one with your hands is the essence of shiatzu. Whether you are giving to another or practicing self-shiatzu, energy is transmitted from your hands.

Specifically, shiatzu is given with the thumbs, fingers and palms, but these serve only as the outlet for your energy. In fact, you give shiatzu with your entire body, focusing your weight and consciousness at your fingers.

When giving shiatzu to a partner, you soon develop an ability to sense the degree of pressure which should be exerted. You should be on the thin line between pleasure and mild pain. The more tension you sense, the greater the pressure you should offer.

One way to become familiar with the various pressures is to practice your touch on a bathroom scale. Place the flats, or the bulbs, of both of your thumbs on the scale. Straighten your arms and press straight down with your arms bearing your body weight until the scale indicator reaches twenty pounds. This is the amount of maximum pressure which should be applied to the strong-muscled portions of the body. Count to three and raise your thumbs from the scale, pause, and again press down for a three count. Repeat this a few times until you are familiar with the amount of pressure which you must exert to reach the twenty-pound level. Do the same exercise at fifteen pounds and at ten pounds. Fifteen pounds is approximately the pressure you should use on the head and

Chapter 2

Touch

stomach. Ten pounds is the level for the front and sides of the neck and the lower abdomen.

GIVING SHIATZU TO A PARTNER

The only equipment you need when giving shiatzu is a blanket or quilt, a towel or small pillow, and a floor or bed. I prefer using the floor rather than a bed or massage table. It allows me more freedom to take positions above the head, and from side to side, and at the feet.

You can make a pallet by folding one or two blankets in thirds, lengthwise on the floor. Since small hard pillows are seldom available in homes, you can create an excellent headrest by folding a towel several times, until it is approximately two inches thick. This will serve as a rest for the head when your partner is on the stomach and a neck support when she is on the back.

It is important that when you press on your partner you do so with arms extended. The weight behind your pressure should be centered in your shoulders and back. This makes it possible for your touch to be as direct and focused as possible. It also dictates the position which you must be in.

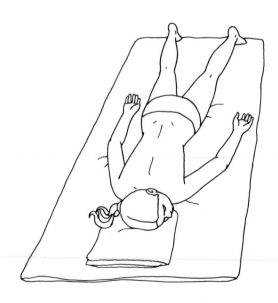

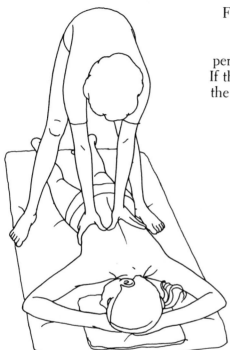

For instance, when working on the spine you should be straddling your partner. Your arms should be as close to a perpendicular line to the spine as possible. If this becomes too tiring, you can kneel at the side and position your upper body over the area you are concentrating on.

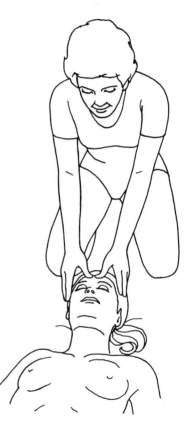

When shiatzu is given to the head, arms and legs the kneeling position is best. Again, you must concentrate on keeping your arms extended and use the weight and balance of your shoulders and upper back.

There are three basic ways of giving shiatzu "touch" to a partner:

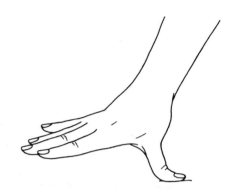

SINGLE THUMB

The most frequently used method is direct pressure from the bulb of the thumb. Try to imagine that the point of contact is at the center of your thumb directly behind the base of your thumbnail. Don't be surprised if you find that your thumb becomes a bit sore the first few times you try. As with everything physical you'll be undergoing a conditioning of your own. You'll soon become used to it.

THUMBS SIDE BY SIDE

When pressing areas where you want a wider touch, i.e., near the spine, you should use both thumbs. They should be touching and form an angle to each other of approximately forty-five degrees. Use the complete bulb of each thumb. Side-by-side thumb pressure is also used on the top of the head and on the back and sides of the legs and arms.

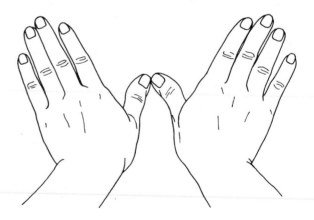

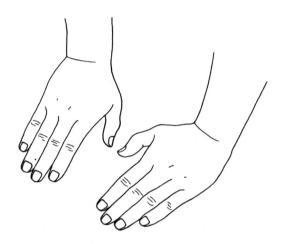

PALMS

An excellent method for the broad portions of the lower back, the stomach and the abdomen is to press with your flattened palms. Pressure should be centered in the middle of the hands, and the fingers and palms should also be in contact with your partner.

In the chapters which follow I shall specify which of these three methods should be used on each part of the body.

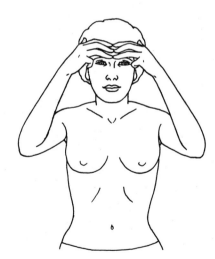

HOW TO GIVE YOURSELF SHIATZU

Self-shiatzu is done best while you are sitting either in a chair or on the floor. Except when working on your lower legs and feet, you will be unable to give self-pressure with your arms extended. You should, however, keep your elbows on the same plane as the direction of the pressure, giving pressure with your entire forearm. When points on the top and side of your head are pressed, your elbows should point outward.

In self-shiatzu you often use single-thumb pressure and

thumbs side by side. The method you will use most frequently is a combination of two or three fingers.

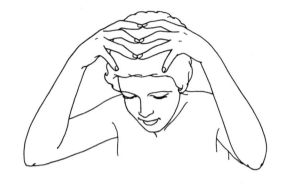

FINGERS SIDE BY SIDE

Using two or three fingers at a time is the easiest method for exerting pressure on yourself. It makes it possible for you to do your back and shoulders. It also increases the size of the pressure area. The fingers should be arched and the contact should be made with the rounded portions of the fingers, not the tips.

With self-shiatzu you will soon discover for yourself how to maximize the effect of your touch. With partner-shiatzu you must work as a team. You must attune yourself to another's needs. A sigh or a groan will often tell as much as any words, and through your hands you will begin to experience the spiritual reward of sharing energy.

Chapter 3

Shiatzu for a Youthful Complexion

Shiatzu will make you look younger by improving the color and the texture of your skin. Virtually everyone to whom I give regular complete shiatzu experiences marked improvement. This, I feel, is a direct result of shiatzu's ability to stimulate the circulatory system and improve muscle tone.

In Oriental medicine beautiful skin tone is considered a reflection of excellent general health—a result of the unity of the body. By opening the meridians, the energy pathways, and improving circulation throughout the body, shiatzu significantly affects the beauty of the skin.

The specific factors which contribute to a glowing complexion are agreed upon both in the Orient and in the West, i.e., proper circulation and muscle tone, hormonal balance, particularly estrogen, adequate sleep, and avoidance of lingering fatigue.

The exercises which I recommend for improved facial tone take only about ten minutes a day. For best and sustained results you should follow the sequence at least four times a week. And you can expect to feel and see results within the first two weeks. My exercises relax muscle tension, maintain the skin's moisture, and improve circulation throughout the neck and face. They are done on the lower back, the abdomen, the ankles and feet, the neck, and the face.

When giving shiatzu specifically for skin beauty I always begin on the lower back. Shiatzu here relieves muscle tension and serves as a stimulant to the adrenal glands and the reproductive organs. It also helps in maintaining a proper hormonal balance.

I then move to the abdomen to aid general circulation. Shiatzu on the abdomen also improves the functions of the liver, the stomach, and the intestines.

Next comes shiatzu on the ankles and feet. This is important, for proper circulation to this area, most distant from the heart, is critical to the effectiveness of the entire circulatory system. In addition, shiatzu on the soles of the feet helps to relax the entire body, and, not unimportantly, it feels wonderful.

Finally, I do the face and neck. Gentle pressures give proper tone to the facial muscles and heighten the flow of blood to the sensitive cells in the several layers of facial skin. In Oriental medicine the neck is known as the Fountain of Beauty and Youth. Shiatzu on the front and sides of the throat and neck helps to keep the major arteries and veins elastic. It also stimulates healthy circulation between the heart and the brain and the face.

I feel that the ideal time for shiatzu for facial beauty is in the morning, while you are readying yourself for the day. If, however, your schedule doesn't allow this, you will get the same results by doing the exercises when they are convenient. The most important thing is that you do the full sequence consistently.

You will probably find that the self-shiatzu version of the exercises is quite easy. I have also detailed a set of partner-shiatzu for facial beauty exercises. Without minimizing the effects of self-shiatzu it is, when possible, more pleasant to have someone else applying the pressures to you.

SELF-SHIATZU FOR THE COMPLEXION

You can do these exercises sitting either in a chair or on the floor. I prefer sitting in a chair for it becomes easier to relax my legs.

Lower Back

Reach behind yourself and place your right thumb three finger-widths out from the center of the spine in the middle of your lower back, as high up as you can reach while maintaining enough leverage for deep (20-pound) pressure. Do the same with your left thumb.

1 Give deep (20-pound) pressure at both points for three seconds. Pause.

2 Move your thumbs down in a straight line halfway to your waist. Repeat the deep pressure. Pause.

3 Move directly down to the waistline, with each thumb still three finger-widths out from the center of the spine. Repeat the deep pressure. Pause.

4 Place your thumbs back up at your starting point. Then move each thumb out to points five finger-widths from the center of the spine. Give deep (20-pound) pressure for three seconds. Pause.

5 Move directly down halfway to the waistline. Repeat the pressure. Pause.

6 Move straight down and place your thumbs on the waistline. Repeat the deep (20-pound) pressure.

Upper Abdomen

The six points on your upper abdomen form an imaginary cross. The first four points lie along the meridian of conception, the vertical line which bisects the stomach from the bottom of the rib cage to just above the navel. The last two points lie below the rib cage, on a line straight down from the center of each breast.

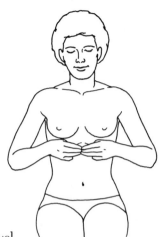

1 Place the index, middle and third fingers of both hands side by side on the first point, just below the center of the rib cage. Give moderate (15-pound) pressure with both hands for three seconds. Pause.

2 Move down three finger-widths toward the navel. Repeat the moderate (15-pound) pressure with both hands for three seconds. Pause.

3 Move three finger-widths further down the line and repeat the moderate pressure. Pause.

4 Move three more finger-widths down the line. You should now be just slightly above the navel. Repeat the moderate (15-pound) pressure. Pause.

5 Separate your hands and do the two points immediately below the rib cage simultaneously. Use the three fingers of each hand on the respective points. Give moderate pressure for three seconds.

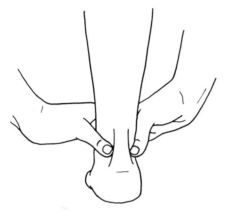

Ankles

Rest your right foot on the floor. Lean forward to work on the ankle. Place your right thumb on the outside of the ankle at the top of the recess between the anklebone and the Achilles tendon, which runs into the back of the heel. Place your left thumb on the corresponding point on the inside of the ankle. Then wrap your fingers around the front of the ankle.

1   Give moderate (15-pound) pressure with both thumbs for three seconds. Pause.

2   Move your thumbs down the inside of the Achilles tendon to the deep recess between the back of the anklebone and the tendon. Repeat the moderate pressure with both thumbs. Pause.

3   Move down to the recess above the top of the heel. Repeat the moderate (15-pound) pressure with both thumbs.

4   Now repeat the same sequence on your left ankle.

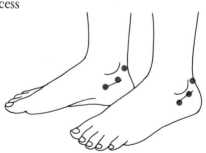

Soles

Place your right leg on your left knee so that you can grip your foot with both hands and press the points on your sole with both thumbs side by side. The first three points to receive pressure are on a line which bisects the foot from heel to toe. The last is high in the rear of the arch, on the inside corner of the heel, above and slightly forward of the first point.

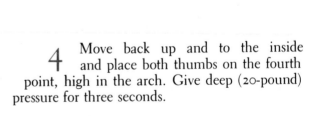

1 Wrap your hands around the top of your foot and place your thumbs side by side just in front of the center of the heel pad. Give deep (20-pound) pressure for three seconds. Pause.

2 Move down the center line to the narrowest part of the foot and repeat the deep pressure. Pause.

3 Move down to the point just behind the ball of the foot. Repeat the deep pressure. Pause.

4 Move back up and to the inside and place both thumbs on the fourth point, high in the arch. Give deep (20-pound) pressure for three seconds.

5 Place your left leg on your right knee and repeat the sequence on your left foot.

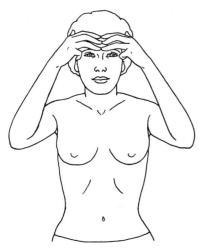

Forehead

In this sequence your fingertips should be perpendicular to your forehead and your hands will move outward from the center of the forehead to your temples.

1   Touch the tips of your index fingers together just below the center of your hairline—on the widow's peak. Touch the tips of your middle fingers together in the center of your forehead. Your third fingers should fall directly below the middle fingers just above the space between the eyebrows.

2   Give moderate (15-pound) pressure with the index, middle, and third fingers of both hands simultaneously. Pause. Repeat the pressure two more times.

3   Move your fingers apart and out to the points which run from the hairline to the centers of the eyebrows. Repeat the moderate pressure with the fingers of both hands simultaneously. Pause. Repeat two more times.

4   Move your hands out to the points which run from the hairline to the ends of the eyebrows. Repeat the moderate pressure with all of the fingers simultaneously. Hold for three seconds. Repeat the pressure two more times.

Eyes

The points surrounding the eyes are on the inside edges of the eye sockets. Use the index, middle and third fingers of both hands—the left hand for the left eye and the right hand for the right eye. Do both eyes simultaneously. If you are wearing contact lenses remove them.

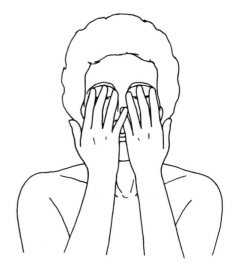

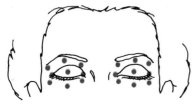

1 Spread your fingers slightly and place the bulbs on the inside of the upper ridges of the eye sockets, with the third finger of each hand as close to the nose as possible. With the fingers brushing lightly over your closed eyes, press upward against the inner ridge of the sockets with light (10-pound) pressure for three seconds.

2 Draw your fingers down slightly, with the bulbs resting on your closed eyelids. Press gently (2–3 pounds) for three seconds.

3 Arch your fingers slightly and press on the inner edge of the lower ridges of the eye sockets. Use light (10-pound) pressure against the bone for three seconds.

Nose

Place the bulbs of your middle fingers on the nails of your index fingers. Press corresponding points on both sides of the nose simultaneously.

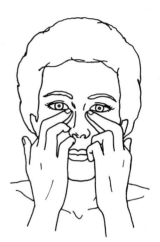

1 Place your right fingers on the right where the side of the nose joins the cheekbone, slightly below the tear ducts. Place your left fingers on the corresponding point on the left side of the nose. Give moderate (15-pound) pressure for three seconds. Pause.

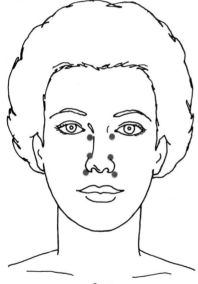

2 Move your fingers down to the middle of the sides of the nose, on the cheek/nose line, just above the flares of the nostrils. Repeat the pressure. Pause.

3 Move down to the bottom of the sides of the nose at the corners of the nostrils. Repeat the moderate (15-pound) pressure. Hold for three seconds.

Cheeks

Keep the tips of your middle fingers on top of the nails of your index fingers. There are four points on each cheek. Press the corresponding points on the right and left cheeks simultaneously.

1 The first pair of points is directly below the centers of the eyes, one finger-width down from the center of the lower ridge of the eye sockets. Give moderate (15-pound) pressure for three seconds. Pause.

2 Move two finger-widths out toward the sides of the face to the high point of the cheekbones, slightly below the outer corners of the eyes. Repeat the moderate (15-pound) pressure for three seconds. Pause.

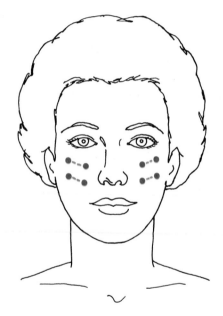

3 Move your fingers back to the points directly below the initial points, on a line with the bottom of the nose. Give moderate pressure for three seconds. Pause.

4 Move your fingers two finger-widths out toward the sides of the face, and one finger-width below the high point of the cheekbones. Repeat the moderate (15-pound) pressure. Hold for three seconds.

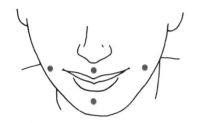

Mouth

There are four points near the mouth. Use one of your thumbs for the first and last points and both thumbs simultaneously for the second and third.

1   Place your thumb at the point midway between the nose and the upper lip. Give moderate (15-pound) pressure for three seconds. Pause.

2   Place each thumb two finger-widths beyond the corners of the mouth. Give moderate pressure for three seconds. Pause.

3   Place your thumb midway between the center of the lower lip and the tip of the chin. Give moderate (15-pound) pressure for three seconds.

Under Chin

The point under the chin is in the recessed area two finger-widths behind the front of the jawbone. Reach under with the bulb of your thumb.

1   Give moderate (15-pound) pressure for three seconds. Pause.

2   Repeat the pressure.

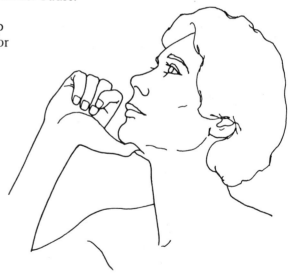

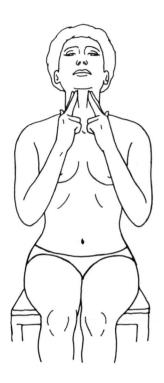

Neck and Throat

For the points on the neck, use the index and middle fingers of both hands, the left hand for the left side of the neck and the right hand for the right side. The points shown in the illustration are for general guidance. The idea is to cover the neck area with light to moderate pressure. Do corresponding points on both sides at the same time.

1 Place the index and middle fingers of your right hand under your jaw at the side of the top of the windpipe. Do the same on the left side with your left hand. Give light (10-pound) pressure for two seconds, into the muscle, not the windpipe. Pause.

2 Move your fingers down slightly and repeat the pressure.

3 Continue down the line to the base of the neck, giving light pressure at each point for two seconds.

4 Bring your hands back up to the top of the neck and repeat the pressures. Trace the major neck muscles from the top to the base of the neck.

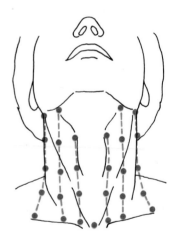

There is a single point at the base of the neck, between the collarbones. Bend your thumb and place the tip on the top of the bone. Press down toward the feet, not into the throat. Give moderate (15-pound) pressure for three seconds. Pause. Repeat twice more.

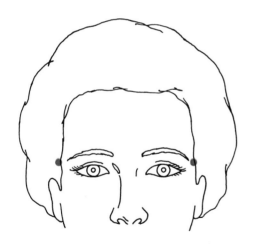

Temples

With the points on the temples, the self-shiatzu sequence is completed. Cross the tips of your middle fingers over the nails of the index fingers.

1 Locate the slight recesses at the temples. With both hands simultaneously, give moderate (15-pound) pressure for three seconds. Pause.

2 Repeat the pressure. Hold for three seconds.

Rest for a few moments when you finish this self-shiatzu. Sit back in your chair and inhale through your nose, filling your lungs with air. Hold the air for three seconds and then exhale slowly through your mouth. Repeat this at least six times.

PARTNER-SHIATZU FOR THE COMPLEXION

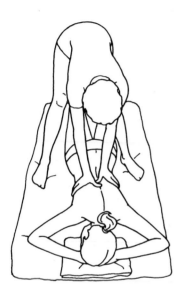

Spine

Your partner should be lying face down on the floor on a folded blanket or pallet, her head resting on her hands on a small stiff pillow or folded towel. Straddle your partner, placing your feet on a line slightly below her hips. Give pressure with your arms extended and the weight of your upper body transmitted down to and through your thumbs.

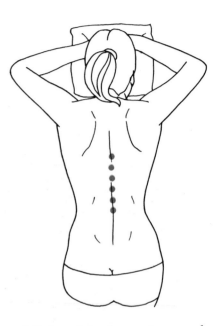

1 With your right thumb locate the recess or ditch between the vertebra below your partner's shoulder blades. Give moderate (15-pound) pressure for three seconds. Pause.

2 Move down the spine and place your left thumb in the next recessed point below the next vertebra. Give moderate (15-pound) pressure for three seconds. Pause.

3 Alternate your thumbs right, then left, following the recessed points to the waistline. Give moderate pressure at each point.

Right and Left Sides of the Spine

1 Place your thumbs side by side midway between the bottom of the shoulder blades and the waistline, two finger-widths to the right of the spine. Give moderate (15-pound) pressure for three seconds. Pause.

2 Move your thumbs down to a point halfway to the waistline. Repeat the pressure. Pause.

3 Move directly down to the waistline and repeat the moderate (15-pound) pressure. Pause.

4 Move back up to a point four finger-widths to the right of the spine, midway between the bottom of the shoulder blade and the waistline. Repeat the previous sequence on the line, ending at the waist.

5 Repeat the sequence on the left side of the spine, first two finger-widths out from the spine, then four finger-widths out from the spine.

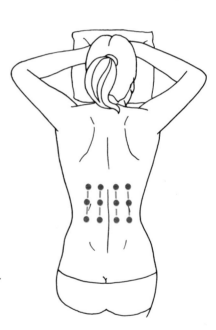

Ankles

Kneel beside your partner's right knee, looking toward the right ankle. Place your right thumb on the inside of the ankle, in the top of the recess between the anklebone and the Achilles tendon. Place your left thumb on the corresponding point at the outside of the ankle. Wrap your fingers around the front of the ankle.

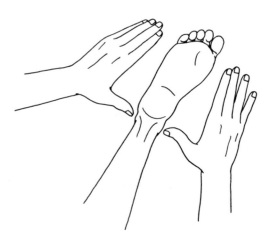

1 Give moderate (15-pound) pressure with both thumbs for three seconds. Pause.

2 Move both thumbs down the inside of the Achilles tendon to the deep recess between the back of the anklebone and the tendon. Repeat the moderate pressure. Pause.

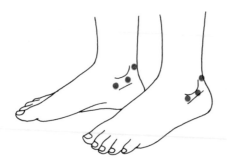

3 Move your thumbs down to the recess above the top of the heel. Repeat the pressure. Hold for three seconds. Pause.

4 Move to your partner's left and repeat the pressures on the left ankle.

Soles

Position yourself below your partner's feet, looking toward her head. The first three points on the sole are on a line bisecting the foot. The fourth and last is high in the arch, above the inside corner of the heel, slightly forward of the first point.

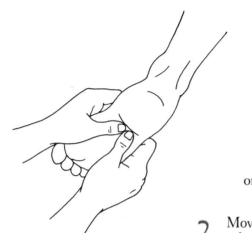

1   Wrap your fingers around the top of your partner's right foot and place your thumbs side by side just below the center of the heel pad. Give deep (20-pound) pressure for three seconds. Pause.

2   Move down the line to the center of the sole. Repeat the pressure for three seconds. Pause.

3   Place your thumbs side by side on the point just behind the ball of the foot. Repeat the pressure. Pause.

4   Move back up and to the inside, and place both thumbs on the fourth point, high in the arch. Give deep (20-pound) pressure for three seconds.

5   Repeat the pressures at the corresponding points on the sole of the left foot.

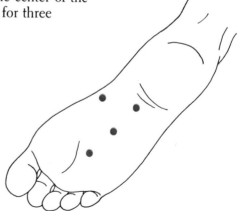

Upper Abdomen

Have your partner change position and rest on her back. Kneel at her right side. You can cover all of the abdomen points from this position. The six points form an imaginary cross right in the center of the stomach area.

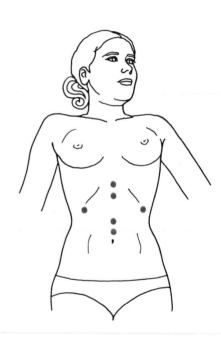

1 Place both thumbs together just below the bottom center of the rib cage. Give moderate (15-pound) pressure. Hold for three seconds. Pause.

2 Move down two finger-widths. Give moderate (15-pound) pressure. Hold for three seconds, then pause.

3 Move three finger-widths further down the line and repeat the moderate (15-pound) pressure. Pause.

4 Move down to the point just slightly above the navel. Repeat the moderate (15-pound) pressure. Pause.

5 Move back up to the point below the bottom rib on the right side on a line with the nipple. Give moderate (15-pound) pressure with both thumbs. Hold the pressure for three seconds, then pause.

6 Move to the left rib point and repeat the pressure.

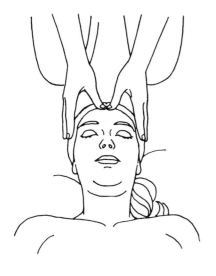

Forehead

Kneel above your partner's head. You should be able to reach the top of her head without stretching. The points on the forehead run down five lines between the hairline and the line of the eyebrows. The first line runs down the center of the forehead. The second and third (a pair) run from the hairline through the middle of each of the eyebrows. The fourth and fifth (another pair) run from the hairline down to the outside ends of the eyebrows.

1   Place your thumbs side by side at the widow's peak. Give moderate (15-pound) pressure for three seconds. Pause.

2   Move the thumbs two finger-widths down the line toward the nose. Repeat the pressure. Pause.

3   Move to the point between the eyebrows and repeat the moderate pressure. Pause.

4   Separate your thumbs and move them back to the hairline at the beginning of the lines that run down to the middle of the eyebrows. Give moderate (15-pound) pressure for three seconds. Pause.

5   Move down these lines at two finger-width intervals, ending at the points at the center of the eyebrows.

6   Move your thumbs back to the hairline at the top of the two outside lines. Move down these lines at two finger-width intervals. Give moderate pressure at each point, ending at the outer edges of the eyebrows.

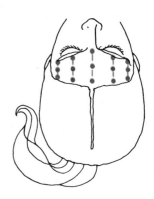

Eyes

The points surrounding the eyes are on the inside edge of the eye sockets. Use your index fingers and give pressure to corresponding points on the right and left eyes simultaneously.

1 Place your index fingers on the inner edge of the upper ridges of the eye sockets, as close to the nose as possible. Give light (10-pound) pressure directly on the inner edge of the sockets. Hold the pressure for three seconds. Pause.

2 Move your fingers one finger-width along the bone toward the outside of the sockets. Repeat the pressure. Be sure to keep the bulbs of your fingers directly on the inner edges of the sockets. Pause.

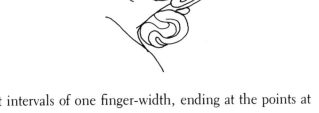

3 Continue the pressures at intervals of one finger-width, ending at the points at the outside of the sockets.

4 Press the flats of your index and middle fingers lightly (2–3 pounds) onto the closed eyelids. Hold this gentle pressure for three seconds.

You will have to change your position to reach the lower ridges of the eye sockets. Kneel beside your partner's midsection. Use your index fingers simultaneously on the corresponding points of the right and left eyes.

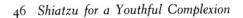

1 Starting as close to the nose as possible, give light (10-pound) pressure directly down on the inner edge of the sockets. Hold the pressure for three seconds. Pause.

2 Move your fingers one finger-width along the lower edges of the sockets. Repeat the pressure. Pause.

3 Continue the pressures at intervals of one finger-width, ending at the points at the outside edges of the sockets.

Nose

Return to your kneeling position above your partner's head. To give shiatzu to the points at the sides of the nose, place the balls of your middle fingers on the nails of your index fingers. Press corresponding points on both sides of the nose simultaneously, with the tips of the index fingers.

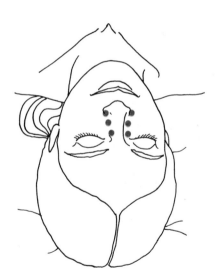

1 Place your fingers at the sides of the nose, slightly below the bridge, where the cheekbone meets the nose. Give moderate (15-pound) pressure for three seconds. Pause.

2 Move down the cheek/nose line to the outside middle of the nose, just above the flares of the nostrils. Repeat the moderate pressure. Pause.

3 Move down to the bottom of the sides of the nose, at the outside corners of the nostrils. Repeat the moderate (15-pound) pressure.

Cheeks

There are four shiatzu points on each cheek. Use your thumbs on the corresponding points simultaneously.

1 Start with the pair of points directly below the centers of the eyes, one finger-width below the center of the lower ridge of the eye sockets. Give moderate (15-pound) pressure for three seconds. Pause.

2 Move your thumbs out toward the sides of the face. Locate the highest points of the cheekbones, slightly below the outer corners of the eyes. Repeat the moderate pressure for three seconds. Pause.

3 Move your thumbs back two finger-widths below the first points, on a line with the bottom of the nose. Give moderate (15-pound) pressure for three seconds. Pause.

4 Move your thumbs out toward the sides of the face, two finger-widths below the highest points of the cheekbones. Repeat the moderate pressure for three seconds. Pause.

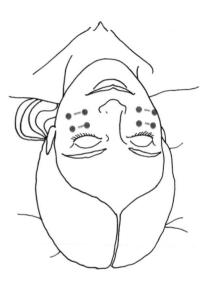

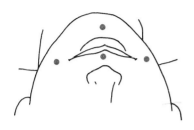

Mouth

There are four points near the mouth. Use one of your thumbs for the first and last points and both thumbs simultaneously for the second and third.

1 Place your thumb midway between the bottom of the nose and the upper lip. Give moderate (15-pound) pressure for three seconds. Pause.

2 Place each thumb two finger-widths beyond the corners of the mouth. Give moderate (15-pound) pressure for three seconds. Pause.

3 Place your thumb in the recess midway between the center of the lower lip and the tip of the chin. Repeat the moderate (15-pound) pressure. Hold for three seconds.

Under Chin

Move to your partner's right side and kneel by her waist.
The point under the chin is located two finger-widths in from the front of the chin. Reach under the chin and locate the point with the tip of your middle finger.

1 Give moderate (15-pound) pressure for three seconds. Pause.

2 Repeat the pressure.

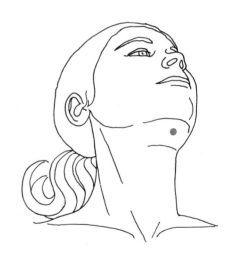

Neck

Remain at the right of your partner's upper body. You should be able to reach the neck comfortably without stretching your arms. Although specific points are shown in the illustration, you need to use them only as a general guide. The idea is to cover the neck area thoroughly. Just cover the general area, starting beneath the jaw and working down to the base of the neck. Use the index and middle finger of both hands, alternating your right and left hands.

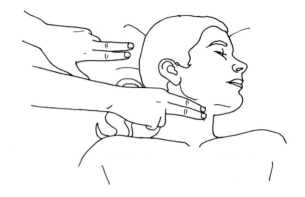

1 Place the index and middle fingers of your right hand under the jaw beside the top of the windpipe. Give light (10-pound) pressure at the top of a line made by the side of the windpipe and the muscle. Be careful not to press directly on the windpipe, but into the muscle. Hold for two seconds. Pause.

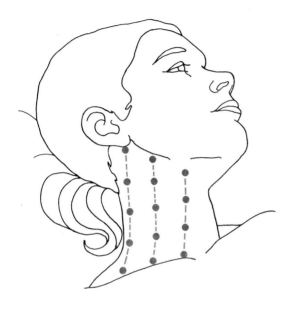

2 Place the index and middle fingers of your left hand just below the point you have just pressed with your right hand. Repeat the light pressure.

3 Continue to move straight down alongside the windpipe, alternating your hands to give light pressure, until you reach the base of the neck.

4 Bring your hands back up to the top of the neck under the jaw. Repeat the pressures, alternating your hands along a descending line to the base of the neck.

5 Continue the light (10-pound) pressures from the top of the neck to the base until you have covered the right side of the neck.

6 Move to your partner's left side and repeat the sequences on the left side of the neck.

Temples

Return to your position above your partner's head. The last points in the series are on the temples. Cross the tips of your middle fingers over the nails of your index fingers.

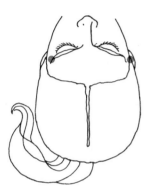

1 Find the slight recesses at the temples. Use both hands simultaneously and give moderate (15-pound) pressure for three seconds. Pause.

2 Repeat the pressure.

Final Exercises

Have your partner extend her arms out on the floor above her head. Grip her hands and pull gently, stretching her arms. At the same time, your partner should inhale through her nose, filling her lungs to capacity, while stretching her legs and toes. Hold a moment, then release the tension on her hands while she exhales slowly through her mouth, relaxing her whole body. Repeat this exercise six times.

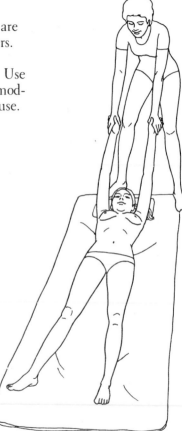

Chapter 4

Shiatzu for Sexual Vigor

Shiatzu can increase your sexual vigor. Through shiatzu, declining sexuality can be revived and sexual awareness, sensitivity and drive can be heightened.

I consider sexuality an important aspect of an individual's unity and Oneness. Often during my years in shiatzu I have seen people, particularly those who lead pressured lives, experience a diminished sexual drive. With shiatzu I helped them regain their sexual energy.

To view the functional role shiatzu can play in sexuality it is necessary to consider the connection between sexuality and physical health. The key to an excellently functioning body rests with relaxed and correctly toned muscles. The muscles of the lower back, abdomen, thighs and neck must be relaxed. Adequate blood circulation is also essential in maximizing sexual energy and heightening sensitivity.

The shiatzu exercises which I have designed for partners will serve you well. Because the brain controls the sexual activities and motor responses, deep pressures are given to the top and the back of the head. The lower back, the lower abdomen and the inner thighs receive steady pressures, to relax the muscles, improve circulation and heighten sensitivity. The neck receives tender pressure in order to relax the abdominal organs and improve the metabolism and circulation between the heart and the brain. The palms of the hands and the soles of the feet are also included to facilitate full body relaxation and heightened sensitivity. The point of the entire sequence is to relax and to stimulate—the words are not contradictory.

Shiatzu for sexual vigor is rewarding for both men and women. In this chapter I describe it from the viewpoint of a woman giving shiatzu to a man. This series is designed to be done comfortably on a bed, although I strongly feel that all other partner-shiatzu series should be done on a floor or firm pallet. In this case a bed is simply more comfortable.

Many people who have regained their sexual vigor through shiatzu have told me that they continue to use the series as a rewarding and sense-heightening form of foreplay. This, of course, it is. And I strongly recommend it for both purposes.

Of all the physiological values of shiatzu in heightening or reawakening sexual drive, I believe that perhaps the greatest benefit of these "exercises" is the wonderfully sensuous feeling that both partners experience from the pressures. It is indeed a form of communicating one's love and caring to another. And whether you are concerned with regaining or increasing sexual energy and activity, shiatzu can and will serve within a period of days to bring both you and your partner closer to a state of Oneness.

Head

Your partner should be lying face down. Since you probably won't have enough room on your bed to position yourself above the top of your partner's head, try sitting astride your partner with your weight on your lower legs.

There are two points on the head. The first is at the center of the top of the crown. The second is at the base of the skull where it meets the top of the neck.

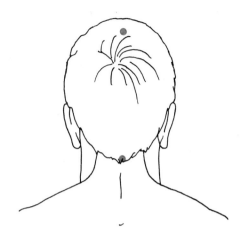

1   Place the index and middle fingers of both your hands on the point at the top of the crown. Give deep (20-pound) pressure for three seconds. Pause.

2   Repeat the pressure. Pause.

3   Repeat the pressure again. Pause.

4   Move your thumbs down to the point at the base of the skull. Place your left thumb on top of the right. Give deep (20-pound) pressure for three seconds. Pause.

5   Repeat the deep pressure two more times.

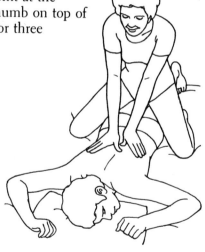

Lower Back

Stay astride your partner and move back until you can comfortably reach the lower part of the spine, from a point just above the waist all the way down to the bottom of the spine.

Run your right thumb down the spine. As you do, you will feel the recesses between the vertebrae. Place your right thumb in one of these recesses slightly above the waistline.

1 Give moderate (15-pound) pressure with your right thumb for three seconds. Pause.

2 Place your left thumb in the next recessed point down the spine. Give moderate pressure for three seconds. Pause.

3 Alternate your thumbs, right, then left, and follow the recessed points down the spine to the end of the tailbone. Give moderate (15-pound) pressure at each point. Then pause and move on.

4 Go back to the point above the waistline and repeat the sequence.

5 Repeat the entire sequence once more.

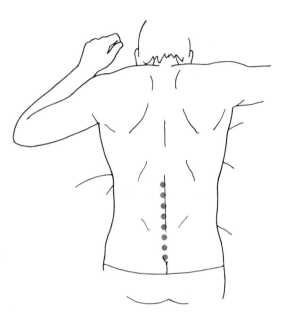

Right and Left Sides of the Spine

Place your thumbs an inch apart on both sides of the spine, slightly above the waistline.

1 Give moderate (15-pound) pressure with both thumbs simultaneously. Pause.

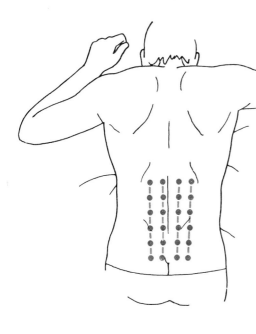

2 Move down the lines two finger-widths and repeat the pressure.

3 Continue down the lines at intervals of two finger-widths. Give moderate (15-pound) pressure with the thumbs at each pair of points for three seconds. Pause for a second after each pressure.

4 Go back to the pair of points slightly above the waistline and repeat the sequence.

5 Repeat the entire sequence again.

6 Place your left thumb an inch and a half to the left of the spine, slightly above the waistline, and the right thumb an inch and a half to the right. Give moderate (15-pound) pressure with both thumbs for three seconds. Pause.

7 Move both thumbs straight down two finger-widths and repeat the pressure. Pause.

8 Continue down the lines at two finger-width intervals until you are on a line with the base of the spine.

9 Repeat the sequence two more times.

Soles

Move back to a position below your partner's right foot. You may have to get off the bed to do this.

There are four points on the sole of each foot which should receive pressure. The first three are on a line which bisects the foot from the center of the heel pad to the center of the ball of the foot. The fourth point is high in the arch, toward the rear, slightly forward of the first point.

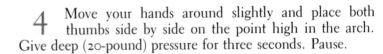

1 Wrap your fingers around the top of the right foot and place both thumbs side by side just in front of the center of the heel pad. Give deep (20-pound) pressure for three seconds. Pause.

2 Move down the line to the center of the narrowest part of the foot. Give deep (20-pound) pressure for three seconds. Pause.

3 Move down the line to the point just behind the center of the ball of the foot. Repeat the deep pressure for three seconds.

4 Move your hands around slightly and place both thumbs side by side on the point high in the arch. Give deep (20-pound) pressure for three seconds. Pause.

5 Repeat the sequence twice more on the sole of the right foot.

6 Move over to a position below your partner's left foot and repeat the sequence three times on the left sole.

Your partner should now turn and lie on his back. The rest of the series proceeds in an irregular pattern. Starting at the right side, you do the right side of the neck, then the abdomen, followed by the right thigh and the right palm. After these sequences you move to your partner's left to do the left side of the neck, the left thigh, and the left palm. The final exercises are special pressures, one for a man, the other for a woman.

Neck

Kneel at the right side of your partner's upper body. Stay close enough so that you can reach the neck without straining. The specific points shown in the neck illustration are only for general guidance. Don't be too concerned with getting the exact points. The idea is to cover the area with light to moderate pressure.

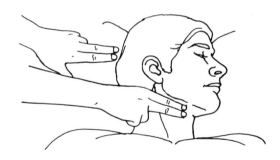

1   Place the index and middle fingers of your right hand under the jaw at the side of the top of the windpipe. Do not press down directly on the windpipe. Instead give light (5- to 10-pound) pressure for three seconds at a point where the neck muscle rests at the edge of the windpipe. Pause.

2   Put your left hand halfway down this line toward the base of the neck and repeat the light pressure. Hold for three seconds. Pause.

3 Move your right hand down to the base of the neck and repeat the light (5- to 10-pound) pressure.

4 Repeat this sequence from the top to the bottom two more times.

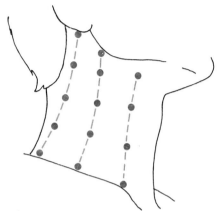

5 Bring your right hand back up to the top of the neck, directly behind the lower back corner of the lower jaw. Give moderate (10- to 15-pound) pressure with the index and middle fingers for three seconds. Pause.

6 Continue down the muscle line at three finger-width intervals, alternating the left hand with the right, until you reach the base of the neck. Give moderate (10- to 15-pound) pressure at each point, holding for three seconds.

7 Repeat the sequence two more times.

8 Bring your right hand back up to a point on the side of the neck directly under the earlobe. Using your index and middle fingers, give moderate (10- to 15-pound) pressure for three seconds.

9 Continue straight down on a line under the earlobe at three finger-width intervals, alternating the left hand with the right, until you reach the shoulder. Give moderate (10- to 15-pound) pressure at each point, holding for three seconds.

10 Repeat this sequence on the side of the neck from the earlobe to the shoulder two more times.

Abdomen

There are three lines of points to press on the abdomen. The first line runs along the meridian of conception, from the center of the breastbone to a point just above the genitals. The second moves outward from the groin along the junction of the legs and trunk. The third follows the line formed by the bottom of the rib cage.

1 Place your thumbs side by side just below the center of the rib cage. Give moderate (15-pound) pressure for two seconds. Pause.

2 Move both thumbs three finger-widths down the center line toward the navel. Repeat the moderate pressure. Pause.

3 Continue down the line to the point just above the genitals. Give moderate (15-pound) pressure for three seconds. Pause.

4 Repeat the pressures (steps 1 to 3) two more times.

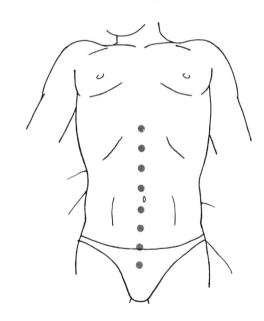

5 Sitting astride your partner's lower legs, place your left thumb at the juncture of the trunk and the top of the inside of the right thigh. Place your right thumb at the corresponding point on the left thigh. Give moderate (15-pound) pressure with both thumbs for two seconds. Pause.

6 Move each thumb two finger-widths along the junction line out toward the sides. Repeat the moderate pressure. Pause.

7 Continue out along the lines at two finger-width intervals until you reach the hips. Give moderate (15-pound) pressure at each point, then pause, and continue.

8 Repeat this sequence (steps 5 to 7) two more times.

9 Place your thumbs under the rib cage, two finger-widths to either side of the center of the body. Give moderate (15-pound) pressure for two seconds. Pause.

10 Move both thumbs two finger-widths out toward the sides, keeping them just under the bottom ribs. Repeat the moderate pressure. Pause.

11 Continue out along the bottom ribs at two finger-width intervals until you reach the sides of the body. Give moderate (15-pound) pressure at each point, pause, then continue.

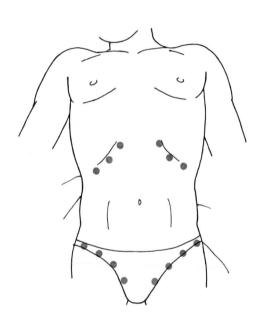

12 Repeat this sequence (steps 8 to 11) two more times.

13 Place both of your hands on the abdomen, palms down, and give light (10-pound) pressure with both palms simultaneously. Move your hands to cover the abdomen with gentle pressure until you feel some relaxation.

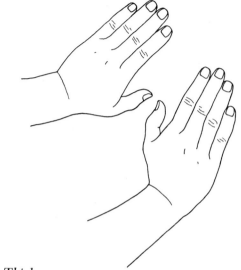

Inside the Thigh

Move to a position next to your partner's right thigh. The points are on a line that begins at the top of the inside of the leg and runs down the center of the inside of the thigh, ending just above the inside of the knee.

1 Place your thumbs side by side at the top of the inside of the leg. Give deep (20-pound) pressure for three seconds. Pause.

2 Move down the muscle line two finger-widths. Repeat the deep pressure. Pause.

3 Repeat the deep pressure at intervals of two finger-widths until you reach the knee.
The last point is in the recess between the knee bone and the tendons at the inside of the knee.

4 Go back to the top of the inside of the leg and repeat the sequence.

5 Repeat the entire sequence once more.

Palm

There are four points on the palm. The first three lie along a line which runs from the base of the wrist to the base of the middle finger. The fourth is at the heel of the thumb.

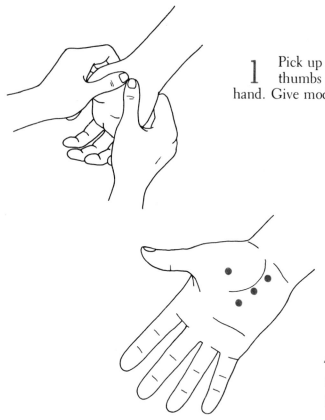

1   Pick up your partner's right hand in both of yours and place your thumbs side by side at the recess in the center of the heel of the hand. Give moderate (15-pound) pressure for three seconds. Pause.

2   Move down the line to the center of the palm. Repeat the moderate pressure. Pause.

3   Place your thumbs on the fleshy pad at the base of the middle finger. Give moderate (15-pound) pressure for three seconds. Pause.

4   Place your thumbs on the point at the heel of the thumb—in the angle formed by the bone leading to the thumb and the bone leading to the index finger. Give moderate pressure for three seconds.

Left Side

Move over to your partner's left side and kneel next to the midsection. Repeat the sequences for the neck, thigh, and palm on your partner's left.

Final Special Pressures

On Men

Locate the point in the center of the perineum, midway between the scrotum and the anus. Press gently three times.

On Women

1 Take a position above your partner's head. Place both your thumbs side by side at the top of the breastbone. Give moderate (15-pound) pressure for three seconds. Then pause.

2 Move two finger-widths down the bone and repeat the pressure.

3 Continue down the bone to the base, just above the top of the stomach. Then repeat the sequence two times.

4 Rest your hands on your partner's breasts with your palms gently touching the nipples. Make slow, gentle circles, rotating the right hand clockwise and the left hand counterclockwise. Make five circles, then pause.

5 Repeat this sequence three more times.

Final Touch

After you finish the shiatzu pressures, you can complete the experience with a special "butterfly touch." Have your partner turn over and rest on the stomach. Using a feather-light touch with the tips of your fingers, draw your fingers over the back of the neck, the back, buttocks, thighs, calves and the soles of the feet in long, flowing caresses. Have your partner turn over again and lie on the back while you give this feathery touch to the neck, chest, abdomen, thighs, shins, arms, and palms. The effect is electrifying, particularly after the shiatzu experience, when the body and mind are relaxed and the blood is flowing freely.

Chapter 5

How to Give Yourself a Complete Shiatzu Experience

Shiatzu is primarily a means of maintaining your health, vitality and serenity. Its true purpose is to prevent problems rather than to remedy them (although I show you how to do the latter later on in this book). One of the keys, perhaps the major key, to gaining shiatzu's fullest benefits is consistent use. The full body self-shiatzu sequences which I have developed should be done, ideally, three or four times a week. The flexibility of self-treatment makes it easy to experience shiatzu regularly. You can apply it to yourself in a relatively short time (the whole sequence as described here takes only fifteen or twenty minutes) and you can give it to yourself wherever you are.

I consider self-shiatzu to be a form of meditative exercise; you will find that one of its great benefits is the sense of calm and inner peace it engenders. I experience it daily, usually at the end of my workday. It affords me a few minutes of quiet and relaxation and it improves my ability to get the most out of the evening. You might prefer to experience shiatzu in the morning, on first arising. You will find it helps you to go through a day at the top of your capacity. And whether you use self-shiatzu in the morning, during the day or in the evening, I'm certain that it will be a help in gaining full and relaxed sleep at the end of the day.

Before you begin this self-shiatzu sequence glance back at Chapter 2, "Touch." Review the positions of the hands and fingers for giving yourself shiatzu. As you repeat the following sequences you will develop your own technique and rhythm. You will also be adding greatly to your ability to give shiatzu to others, for you will learn the locations of the pressure points and the degree of pressure that is most effective.

One of the first things you will discover about your body is that you have several specific points which are extremely tender and responsive to your touch. These eight major points are on the tops of the shoulders, at the top of the shoulder blades, at the center of the shoulder blades, in the armpits, in the valleys of the thumbs, above the buttocks, at the points of the elbows and the insides of the knees. I call these "Yipe" points, for deep shiatzu pressure directly on the points often causes an exclamation. These points are important, for they are areas where large arteries and clusters of nerves serve as major floodgates on the shiatzu pathways.

You will also discover a number of random points which, although less responsive than the "Yipe" points, feel tender or slightly sore to your deep touch. This is to be expected. The tenderness is an indication that your circulation and muscle tone at these points is affected by tensions. Although you are, as a rule, unaware of this interior tenderness, its very real existence indicates specific areas which can benefit greatly from consistent shiatzu. When you locate this type of tenderness or soreness while giving yourself shiatzu, repeat the suggested pressures on the points two or three extra times.

When giving yourself shiatzu don't become too concerned about the precise location of the indicated points. Just remember that your thumb or fingers cover a fairly large area, and inevitably your touch will have the desired effect so long as it is applied firmly in the immediate general vicinity of a given point.

These self-shiatzu exercises can be done while you are sitting, either in a chair or on the floor. Personally, I prefer sitting in a straight-backed chair. It makes it possible to more fully relax my legs. And, unless you're doing shiatzu where you are subject to interruptions, wear as few clothes as you are comfortable with.

Sit down so that both your feet are flat on the floor, your weight is centered on your buttocks, and your back is straight. Relax, take a deep breath, and begin.

HEAD AND NECK

Base of the Skull

Reach both of your hands behind your head to the base of your skull. With the index and middle fingers of both hands, locate the slight indentation at the top center of the neck, just below the base of the skull. In Oriental medicine this point is known as the "Silent Gate."

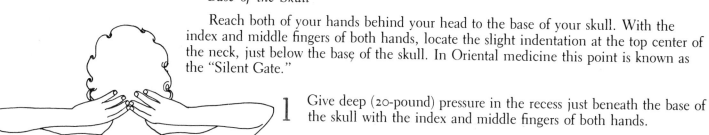

1 Give deep (20-pound) pressure in the recess just beneath the base of the skull with the index and middle fingers of both hands.

2 Hold for three seconds. Pause.

3 Repeat the pressure. Pause.

4 Repeat the pressure.

Neck Muscles

Move your hands apart and place your fingers at the top of the large muscles which run down the outside back of the neck from the base of the skull to the shoulder line. Place your left index and middle fingers at the top of the left muscle where it joins the skull and place the bulbs of your right index and middle fingers at the top of the right muscle. These muscle lines are known as the "Pillars of Heaven." Together with the "Silent Gate" they are important in stimulating circulation to the head and brain.

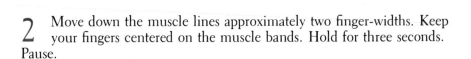

1 Give deep (20-pound) pressure on both points simultaneously for three seconds. Pause.

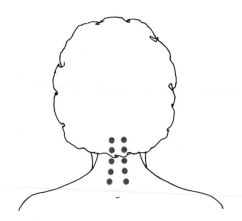

2 Move down the muscle lines approximately two finger-widths. Keep your fingers centered on the muscle bands. Hold for three seconds. Pause.

3 Continue down these neck muscles giving deep (20-pound) pressure at two finger-width intervals. The final points are at the base of the muscles, on the shoulder line.

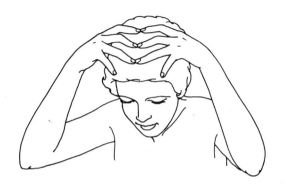

Top of the Head

You give self-shiatsu to the top of your head with the index, middle and third fingers of both hands. Imagine your hair is parted in the middle from hairline to crown. Arch your fingers and place the tips of your middle fingers side by side in the middle of the parting. Then spread the index and third fingers of each hand two finger-widths apart on the same line.

1 Give moderate (15-pound) pressure at the three points simultaneously. Hold for three seconds. Pause.

2 Move your hands apart, out two finger-widths toward the sides of your head. Place the tips of the index, middle and third fingers in line with the initial pressure points. Give moderate (15-pound) pressure for three seconds. Pause.

3 Move each finger out two more finger-widths toward the sides. Repeat the moderate pressure. Hold for three seconds.

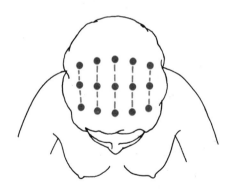

SHOULDERS AND BACK

Shoulders

Locate the point on top of your right shoulder with the index and middle finger of your left hand. The point is halfway between the base of the neck and the edge of your shoulder, slightly to the rear of the central shoulder muscle. This is a "Yipe" point and is called the "Well of the Shoulder." It is a key point where tension often builds up.

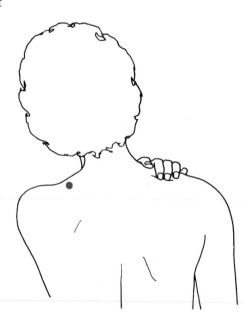

1 Probe with your fingers and locate this central point. When you are on the most tender spot, you have found it.

2 Give deep (20-pound) pressure with the index and middle fingers for three seconds. Pause.

3 Repeat the pressure. Pause.

4 Give pressure again for three seconds. Pause.

5 Locate the corresponding point on your left shoulder with the fingers of your right hand. Repeat the sequence.

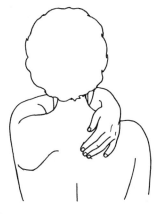

Upper Back

Giving self-shiatzu to your upper back requires some stretching, which is also beneficial. To begin, reach your left hand over your right shoulder. Touch your spine with your index, middle and third fingers, stretching your arm and straightening your back so you are as low on the spine as possible. Then move your fingers one finger-width out from the spine. The initial points run along a line from this point directly up to your shoulder line.

1   Give deep (20-pound) pressure with the index, middle, and third fingers of your left hand. Hold for three seconds. Pause.

2   Move two finger-widths up on a line toward the shoulder. Repeat the deep (20-pound) pressure for three seconds. Pause.

3   Continue giving deep pressure at two finger-width intervals up this line, to and including the final point on the shoulder line.

4   Again extend your left hand as far down the spine as you can reach. Move three finger-widths out from the spine.

5   Give deep pressure for three seconds. Pause.

6   Follow a line directly up to the shoulder at two finger-width intervals. Give deep pressure at each point for three seconds.

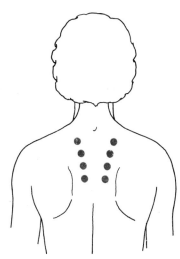

7 The final point is at the shoulder line three finger-widths out from the spine.

8 Switch hands, reaching your right over your left shoulder. Repeat the sequences on the left side of the spine.

Lower Back

Sit forward slightly in your chair. Place your fingertips on the tops of your hipbones and extend your thumbs in toward the spine at the waistline. Place each thumb three finger-widths out from the center of the spine, directly on the waistline.

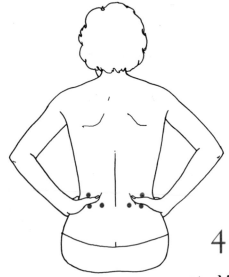

1 Give deep (20-pound) pressure with your thumbs for three seconds. Pause.

2 Repeat the deep pressure. Hold for three seconds. Pause. Repeat the pressure again for three seconds.

3 Move your thumbs directly down three finger-widths. Give deep (20-pound) pressure for three seconds. Pause. Repeat the pressure two more times.

4 Move each of your thumbs three more finger-widths out from the spine. Give deep pressure for three seconds. Pause. Repeat the pressure. Pause. Repeat again.

5 Move your thumbs back up to your waistline. Each thumb should be approximately six finger-widths out from the spine. Give three three-second deep pressures.

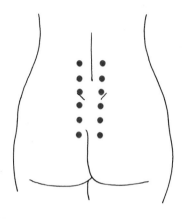

Base of the Spine

You must stand up to do your tailbone. Locate the bottom of the spine (the coccyx) with one hand.

1 With the index and middle fingers of both hands, give moderate (15-pound) pressure. Hold for two seconds. Pause.

2 Move two finger-widths up the bone. Give moderate pressure with both hands for two seconds. Pause.

3 Continue up at intervals of two finger-widths until you reach your waistline.

FACE AND NECK

Forehead

Sit down again to do the rest of the exercises.

In working on your forehead you will move outward from the center of the forehead toward the temples. Remember to keep your elbows on the same plane as the direction of the pressure. They should be raised and pointed outward, the angle increasing as your fingers move toward the temples.

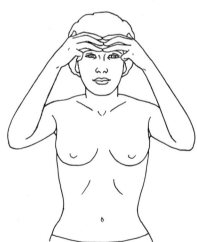

1 Touch the tips of your index fingers together just below the center of your hairline—on the widow's peak, if you have one. Place the tips of your middle fingers directly below them in the center of your forehead; your third fingers should fall directly below the middle fingers, just above the space between the eyebrows.

2 Give moderate (15-pound) pressure with the index, middle and third fingers of both hands simultaneously. Hold for three seconds. Pause.

3 Repeat the moderate pressure for three seconds. Pause.

4 Repeat the pressure. Pause.

5 Move your fingertips out onto the lines which run from the center of each of your eyebrows to the hairline. Give moderate (15-pound) pressure at the three points (top, middle and base) of these lines for three seconds.

6 Repeat the pressure two more times.

7 Move your fingers out onto the set of points running from the hairline to the ends of the eyebrows. Give moderate (15-pound) pressure for three seconds. Pause. Repeat two more times.

8 Using one of your thumbs, press in at the recess above the bridge of your nose. Give deep (20-pound) pressure. Hold for three seconds.

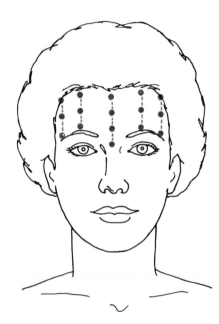

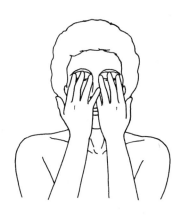

Eyes

The points surrounding the eyes are on the inside edge of the eye sockets. Use the index, middle and third fingers of the left hand for the points indicated for the left eye, and the index, middle and third fingers of the right hand for the right eye. Do both eyes simultaneously. If you are wearing contact lenses, remove them.

1   Spread your fingers slightly and place the bulbs on the inside of the eye sockets' upper ridges. The third finger of each hand should be as close to the nose as possible. With your fingers brushing lightly over your closed eyes press the tips upward against the inner edge of the sockets.

2   Give light (10-pound) pressure for three seconds.

3   Draw your fingers down slightly, resting the bulbs on your closed eyelids. Press gently (2 to 3 pounds) for three seconds. Pause.

4   Arch your fingers slightly and press on the inner edge of the lower ridge of the eye sockets. Use light (10-pound) pressure against the bone for three seconds.

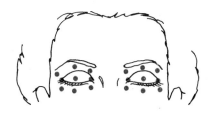

Temples

The points on the temples are slight recesses. Use the index and middle fingers of each hand. Do both the right and left sides simultaneously.

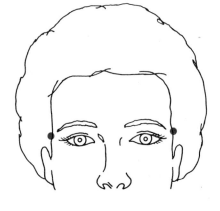

1 Give moderate (15-pound) pressure for three seconds. Pause.

2 Repeat the moderate pressure. Hold for three seconds. Pause.

Cheeks

You give pressure to the points on the cheekbones with your index and middle fingers side by side. Do both the right and left sides at the same time.

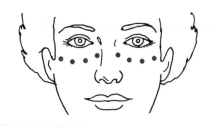

1 Give moderate (15-pound) pressure at the outside edge of the nose, slightly below the bridge of the nose. Hold for three seconds. Pause.

2 Move your fingers out one finger-width onto the flat of the cheekbones. Give moderate (15-pound) pressure for three seconds. Pause.

3 Move two more finger-widths out on the cheekbones. Give moderate pressure for three seconds. Pause.

4 Move one more finger-width out on the cheek. Hold moderate pressure for three seconds. Pause.

Mouth and Chin

There are four points around the mouth.

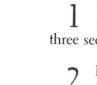

1 Use your right thumb. Give moderate (15-pound) pressure on a point midway between the bottom of the nose and the upper lip. Hold for three seconds. Pause.

2 Place your right thumb on the right cheek point two finger-widths out from the corner of the mouth, with your left thumb on the same spot on the left cheek. Give moderate (15-pound) pressure for three seconds. Pause.

3 Place your right middle fingertip on top of the nail of your right index finger. Give moderate (15-pound) pressure on the chin point midway between the lower lip and the tip of the chin. Hold for three seconds. Pause.

Under Chin

The point under the chin is just behind the front of the lower jawbone. Reach under with the bulb of your right thumb, two finger-widths in from the tip of the chin.

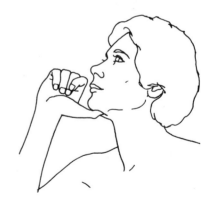

1 Give moderate (15-pound) pressure for three seconds. Pause.

2 Repeat the pressure. Pause.

Neck and Throat

Place the middle finger of your right hand on top of the nail of your right index finger. Place your fingers at the point at the base of the neck where your right and left collarbones join.

1 Give moderate (15-pound) pressure down against the bone, not into your throat. Hold for three seconds. Pause.

2 Repeat the pressure two more times. Hold for three seconds each time.

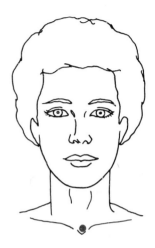

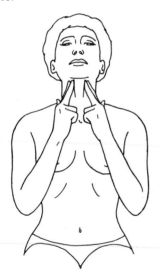

Front and Sides of the Neck

You use the index and middle fingers of both hands on the neck. Although specific points are shown in the illustration, you need to use them only for general guidance. Ideally, you should cover the neck area, using light to moderate pressure. Do the corresponding points on both the right and left sides at the same time.

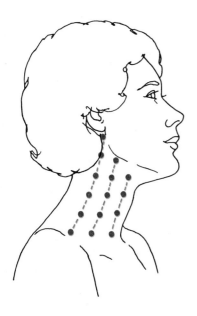

1 Place the index and middle fingers of your right hand under your
   jaw at the side of the top of the windpipe. Take the same
position on the left side with your left hand. Give light (10-pound)
pressure for two seconds at these points. Press down into the muscle, not
onto the windpipe. Pause.

2 Move your fingers down slightly and continue giving light
   pressures for two seconds along the line to the base of the neck.
In Oriental medicine this area is known as the "Fountain of Beauty and
Youth."

3 Bring your hands back to the top of the neck underneath the jaw
   slightly further along the jawline to the side of the neck. Repeat
the pressures on both sides of the neck along a descending line to the
base.

4 Continue the pressures from the top of the neck to the base,
   starting each time further out to the sides of the neck, until you
have covered the front and sides of the neck.

LEGS AND FEET

The sequences which follow take you down the right leg to the sole of the right
foot. When you finish, repeat the sequence on the left leg.

Front of the Thigh

These points go right down the center of the thigh from the groin to the knee.

1   Place your thumb tips side by side in the center of the very top of the leg. Wrap your fingers lightly around the sides of the leg.

2   Give deep (20-pound) pressure for three seconds. Pause.

3   Move your thumbs two finger-widths toward the knee. Give deep pressure for three seconds. Pause.

4   Continue down the line to the top of the kneecap at two finger-width intervals.

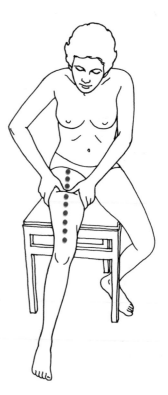

Inside of the Thigh

These points run down the center of the inside thigh. The line begins at the inside of the crotch and traces down to the inside of the knee.

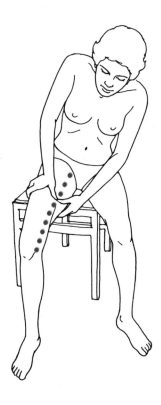

1 Place both thumbs side by side at the uppermost point. The fingers of your left hand should be extended around the underside of your leg. The fingers of your right hand should be extended around the upper portion.

2 Give deep (20-pound) pressure. Hold for three seconds. Pause.

3 Move your thumbs two finger-widths along the bisecting line toward the knee. Give deep (20-pound) pressure for three seconds. Pause.

4 Continue at two finger-width intervals down to the knee.

Lower Leg

The points on the shin are located on lines running down both sides of the leg bone. The first line traces the outside front edge of the bone. The second line runs down along the inside edge of the bone from the knee to the top of the ankle. Cover the points along the outside front edge of the bone first.

1   Place both thumbs side by side right below the bump just below the kneecap on the outside of the shinbone. Wrap your fingers around the leg. Give deep (20-pound) pressure. Hold for three seconds. Pause.

2   Move down two finger-widths and repeat the deep pressure. Hold for three seconds. Pause.

3   Continue down the leg at intervals of two finger-widths. The final point is on the outside edge of the bone at the top of the ankle.

4   Position your thumbs side by side at the top of the inside of the leg bone. Wrap your fingers around your leg and repeat the pressures at two finger-width distances down the leg to the top of the ankle.

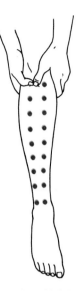

Top of the Foot

The points on the feet are located in the "ditches" between the tendons that lead to the toes. Keep your feet on the floor, lean forward, and place your thumbs side by side in the small ditch approximately two inches back from the apex of the angle formed by the large toe and the first toe.

1   Give moderate (15-pound) pressure for three seconds. Pause.

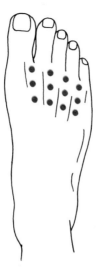

2 Move forward down the ditch halfway to the toes. Give moderate pressure for three seconds. Pause.

3 The third point is right at the end of the ditch. Give moderate pressure for three seconds. Pause.

4 Repeat the sequence in the ditch between each of the bones leading to the toes.

Toes

Rest your right ankle on your left knee. There are points on the top, bottom and side of each of the individual toe bones, midway between the joints.

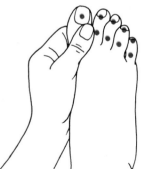

1 Grasp your large toe by placing your left thumb on top of the first bone in the toe, and your index finger directly underneath the opposite. Give moderate (15-pound) squeezing pressure for three seconds. Pause.

2 Move your hand down to the base of the toenail with your thumb still on top and your index finger underneath the toe. Give moderate squeezing pressure for three seconds. Pause.

Self–Shiatzu 85

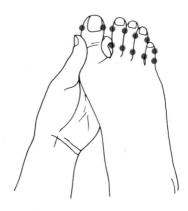

3 Move back to the first bone of the large toe. Give pressure on both sides at the midpoint of the bone by squeezing. Hold for three seconds. Pause. Then repeat the pressure at the sides of the second bone.

4 Give squeezing pressure to each of the toes following the same sequence. Follow along the top and underside of each small bone, then along the sides.

Calf

Place your foot back on the floor. Lean forward and, wrapping your fingers out and around your lower leg, place your thumbs side by side inside the center of the bend of the knee. The points run from the back of the knee to the back of the ankle.

1 Apply deep (20-pound) pressure with your thumbs side by side to the point at the top of the calf muscle. Hold for three seconds. Pause.

2 Move down the center of the muscle two finger-widths. Repeat the deep pressure. Pause.

3 Continue down the muscle at two finger-width intervals. The final pressure point is where the muscle flattens out and joins the top of the ankle.

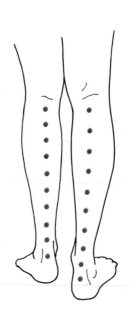

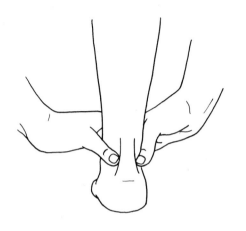

Ankle

Rest your right foot on the floor. Lean forward to work on your ankle. Place your right thumb on the outside of the ankle in the deepest recess between the rear of the anklebone and the Achilles tendon which runs into the back of the heel. Place your left thumb on the corresponding point at the inside of the ankle. Wrap your fingers over your instep.

1   Give moderate (15-pound) pressure with both thumbs for three seconds. Pause.

2   Repeat the pressure for three seconds.

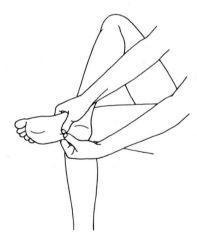

Sole

Rest your right ankle on your left knee. Four points on the sole should receive pressure. The first three are on a line which bisects the foot, one of which is called the "Fountain of Energy." The fourth is high in and to the back of the arch, above and slightly forward of the first point. This point is called the "Valley of the Sole." All four points are effective in helping to alleviate fatigue and to improve circulation throughout the entire body.

1   Grip your foot with both hands and place your thumbs side by side just in front of the heel pad. Give deep (20-pound) pressure for three seconds. Pause.

2   Move down the line to the center (the narrowest part) of the foot. Give deep (20-pound) pressure for three seconds. Pause.

3   The third point is just behind the ball of the foot. Give deep (20-pound) pressure for three seconds. Pause.

4   Shift your hands and place both thumbs side by side on the point high in the arch. Give deep pressure for three seconds.

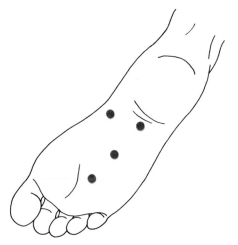

You are now ready to work on your left leg and foot. Go back to the beginning of the Legs and Feet section, and starting at your thigh, follow the sequence down to the sole of your left foot.

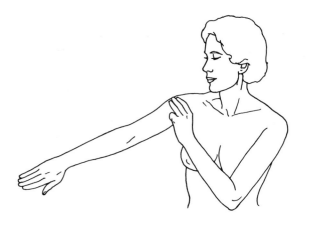

ARMS AND HANDS

Upper Arm

Use your left hand to give shiatzu to your right arm. Press your thumb deep into your right armpit. Extend your fingers halfway around the top of the arm and press the index, middle and third fingertips on the far side of the major arm muscle. Give pressure with your thumb and fingers simultaneously. The line you follow with your thumb traces along the inside of the muscle where it runs down the major bone. The fingers follow a corresponding line on the outside of the muscle and bone.

1 Give deep (20-pound) pressure at the armpit for two seconds. Pause. At the same time squeeze in with your fingers on the outside of your shoulder.

2 Move three finger-widths down the arm along the muscle/bone lines. Give deep (20-pound) pressure with your thumb and fingers. Hold for three seconds. Pause.

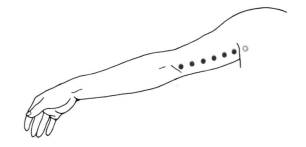

3 Continue down these lines at three finger-width intervals until you reach the elbow. The final points are just above the joint.

Forearm

Roll your right arm so that you are looking down on its outside (back). Place your thumb in the inside of the elbow—in the hollow formed by the bend of the elbow. Extend your fingers over the top of the forearm and grip them on the outside edge of the forearm muscle.

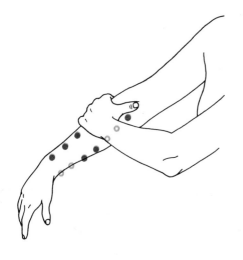

1 Give deep (20-pound) squeezing pressure with your thumb and fingers. Hold for three seconds. Pause.

2 Move down three finger-widths toward the wrist. Keep your thumb on the inside edge of the muscle, your fingers on the outside. Give deep pressure for three seconds. Pause.

3 Continue on to the wrist at intervals of three finger-widths.

Repeat the above sequences on your left upper arm and your left forearm.

Back of the Hand

Spread the fingers of your right hand with the palm facing out. The points are located in the "ditches" between the tendons which run from your wrist to the first knuckles of each of your fingers.

1 Place your left thumb on the mound of muscle above the hollow at the base of the thumb where it joins the hand. Place your left index finger underneath your hand directly

opposite your left thumb. Give deep (20-pound) pressure by squeezing for three seconds. Pause. In Oriental medicine this point is known as the "Valley," and is a "Yipe" point.

2 Move your left thumb to the ditch between your index and middle fingers midway between the wrist and the knuckle. Put your left index finger directly underneath on the palm.

3 Give moderate (15-pound) pressure by squeezing for three seconds. Pause.

4 Moving up the ditch, repeat the pressure at two more points, ending between the knuckles.

5 Press the same three points in the ditches between the tendons leading to the second and third fingers, and then in the ditches between the third finger and the little finger.

6 Repeat the entire sequence on your left hand, using your right thumb and fingers.

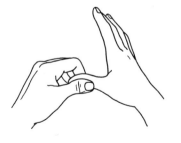

Fingers

Your thumb and each of your fingers should receive pressure at the top, bottom, and sides of each of the individual bones—midway between the joints.

1 Grasp the front and back of the first joint of your right thumb between your left thumb and forefinger. Give moderate (15-pound) squeezing pressure for three seconds.

2 Move your left thumb up to the base of your right thumbnail. Place your left index finger directly opposite. Give moderate (15-pound) squeezing pressure for three seconds.

3 Grasp the sides of the first joint of your right thumb between your left thumb and forefinger. Give moderate (15-pound) pressure for three seconds. Pause.

4 Move thumb and forefinger to the sides of the right thumbnail. Repeat the pressure.

5 Give pressure to each of your fingers in the same manner. Press the first and second joints of each finger, first on top and bottom, then along the sides. Then move on to the next finger.

6 Follow the entire sequence using your right thumb and index fingers on the thumb and fingers of your left hand.

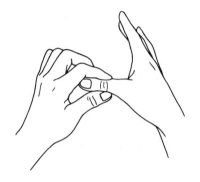

Final Exercises

You can rest for a moment, but you are not quite finished. These final movements are important in maximizing the value of your self-shiatzu.

1   Lie on the floor, flat on your back. Extend your arms up beyond your head.

2   Stretch your arms as far above your head as possible. At the same time, point your toes straight out. Count to five.

3   Still stretching your arms beyond your head, point your toes straight up into the air. Hold for five seconds. Then relax your arms and feet.

4   With your arms still extended, yet relaxed, inhale deeply through your nose. Fill your lungs with air. Hold for a moment and then exhale slowly through your mouth. Repeat this two more times.

5   Relax in this position for at least five minutes before you get up.

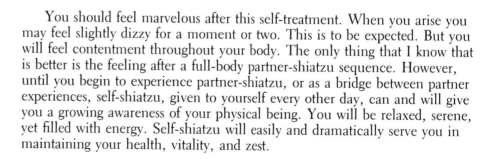

You should feel marvelous after this self-treatment. When you arise you may feel slightly dizzy for a moment or two. This is to be expected. But you will feel contentment throughout your body. The only thing that I know that is better is the feeling after a full-body partner-shiatzu sequence. However, until you begin to experience partner-shiatzu, or as a bridge between partner experiences, self-shiatzu, given to yourself every other day, can and will give you a growing awareness of your physical being. You will be relaxed, serene, yet filled with energy. Self-shiatzu will easily and dramatically serve you in maintaining your health, vitality, and zest.

Full-body partner-shiatzu is shiatzu in its purest and most complete form. A shared experience, it covers the entire body and reaches all of the classical meridians which, viewed as an integrated system, represent the Oneness of being. Both partners are deeply involved, reacting to one another. For the person receiving partner-shiatzu, it is a means to relaxation, well-being, and the staging of renewed energy. To the partner giving shiatzu, it should be a rewarding experience of sharing energy and using one's hands to give physical and emotional well-being.

The instructions for partner-shiatzu are given from the viewpoint of the giver. This is basically what I, as a professional, do during a full-body treatment. To complete the partner sequence will probably take you from forty-five minutes to an hour. Giving full-body shiatzu is physically quite taxing (I take only three patients a day), but you will find that your own physical condition improves as a result of giving partner-shiatzu.

As you gain experience you will discover a language of touch and recognize your ability to communicate with your partner through the tips of your fingers. You will receive messages from your partner, from her reflexive motion, breathing patterns, muscular reactions. As you press certain points on her body she will also react with a yelp of pain. These pain reactions come from proper shiatzu pressure on what I call the "Yipe" points—the eight major points—on the tops of the shoulders, at the top of each shoulder blade, at the center of the shoulder blades, in the armpits, in the valleys of the thumbs, above the buttocks, at the points of the elbows and the insides of the knees. These points are not to be avoided, despite your partner's reaction, for they are critical to shiatzu. They are areas where large arteries and clusters of nerves are located and serve as major floodgates on the shiatzu meridians. Proper

Chapter 6

How to Give Your Partner Full-Body Shiatzu

pressure primes the flow of energy at these points, releasing tensions and accelerating circulation beyond the points.

In giving shiatzu you shouldn't be overly concerned about absolute precision when pressing an indicated point. Just remember that your thumb or fingertip covers a fairly wide area. Invariably your touch will have the desired effect as long as it is applied firmly enough in the immediate general vicinity of a given point.

Before experiencing partner-shiatzu both you and your partner should glance through the instructions in this chapter. You should have an idea in your mind of the general order of shiatzu. Then you are ready to begin. Both you and your partner should wear as few clothes as you are comfortable with. If the room is chilly use a light blanket or bath towel to keep your partner comfortable and covered while you are working on exposed areas of the body.

Your partner should be lying face down on the floor on a folded blanket or pallet, her arms at her sides, her head resting on a small stiff pillow or folded towel. Or she may put her hands on the pillow and rest her head on them. Keep in mind that you are imparting the energy, and throughout partner-shiatzu you must keep your touch tuned to your partner's reactions.

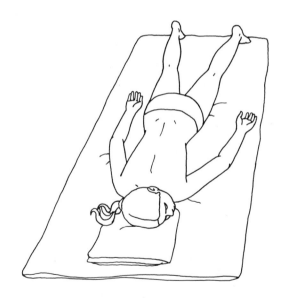

UPPER BODY AND SPINE

Top of the Shoulder

Kneel facing your partner approximately eighteen inches beyond her head. Stay close enough so that you can reach the top of her shoulders easily. Throughout partner-shiatzu you first do the right side, then the left. Extend your left arm, place your thumb on the top of the right shoulder and locate the central point. The back of your hand should be up, your thumb extended beneath. The shoulder point is three or four finger-widths (it depends on the width of your partner's shoulder) out from the base of the neck. It is slightly to the back of the major shoulder muscle. This point is called the "Well of the Shoulder" in Oriental medicine. It is a key point where tension often builds up. And it is one of the "Yipe" points. You will probably hear from your partner when you locate it.

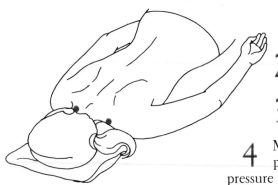

1 Place your right thumbtip on top of your left thumbnail. Give deep (20-pound) pressure for three seconds. Pause.

2 Repeat the deep pressure for three seconds. Pause.

3 Repeat the deep (20-pound) pressure again for three seconds. Pause.

4 Move slightly and line up above your partner's left shoulder. Reverse the position of your thumbs, placing the left on top of the right. Repeat the pressure sequences on this shoulder.

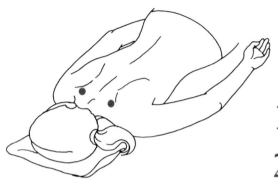

Back of the Shoulder

Remain in the kneeling position and locate the point at the inside top corner of your partner's right shoulder blade with your left thumb. Probe just above the bone.

1 Place your right thumbtip on top of your left thumbnail.

2 Give deep (20-pound) pressure for three seconds. Pause.

3 Repeat the pressure for three seconds. Pause.

4 Reverse your thumbs, placing your left on top of your right. Follow the same sequence on the corresponding point at the inside corner of the left shoulder blade.

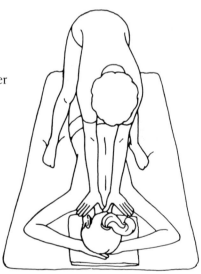

Base of the Skull

You have to shift your position in order to work on your partner's neck. Stand astride her, facing her head, with your feet on a line just below her hips. Bend down from your waist, flex your knees, and with your left thumb on top of your right, place your thumbs slightly below the base of her skull at the top center of her neck. This point is known as the "Silent Gate." It is important in stimulating circulation to the brain.

1 Give deep (20-pound) pressure at this point, just below the base of the skull. Hold the pressure for three seconds. Pause.

2 Repeat the pressure. Pause.

3 Press again for three seconds.

Back of the Neck

Still standing in the same position, spread your thumbs apart and place them at the top of the major muscles which run down the outside back of the neck and join the shoulders. These muscle lines are known as the "Pillars of Heaven." Together with the "Silent Gate" they are important in alleviating headache and tension pains. Place your left thumb at the top of the left muscle where it meets the back of the skull and place your right thumb at the top of the right muscle.

1 Give deep (20-pound) pressure on both points for three seconds. Pause.

2 Move down the muscle lines approximately two finger-widths. Keep your thumbs centered on the muscle bands. Hold for three seconds. Pause.

3 Continue down these neck muscles giving deep (20-pound) pressure at two finger-width intervals. The final point is at the base of the muscles on the shoulder line.

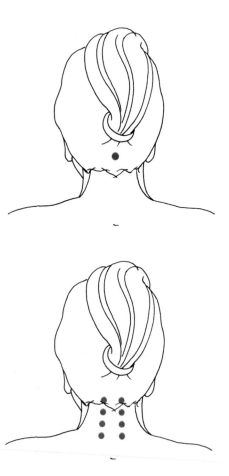

Spine

Now that the head and neck are done, your partner can relax her head and turn and rest the side of her head on the folded towel or pillow. Still straddling, give shiatzu down the entire length of the spine from the base of the neck. If the standing straddle is uncomfortable or tiring, try kneeling astride your partner, resting your weight on your lower legs, not on your partner. In any case, when giving pressure, do it with your arms extended and the weight of your upper body transmitted down to and through your thumbs.

Start at the base of the neck, just beneath the bulging bone—the largest you can feel—at the shoulder line. The spine is, as previously mentioned, the governor meridian and is of extreme importance to your well-being.

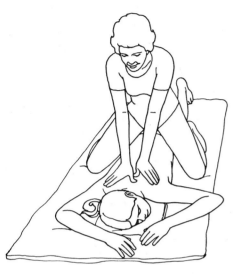

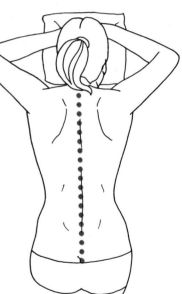

1 Place your right thumb in the recess, or ditch, beneath the bulging bone at the top of the spine where it joins the next vertebra. Give moderate (15-pound) pressure for three seconds. Pause.

2 Move down the spine and place your left thumb on the next recess point. Give moderate (15-pound) pressure for three seconds. Pause.

3 Alternate your thumbs, right, then left, following the recessed points down the spine to the end of the tailbone. Give moderate pressure at each point.

Right and Left Sides of the Spine

1 Moving back to your partner's shoulders, place your left thumb on the shoulder line an inch to the left of the spine, and your right thumb an inch to the right of the spine. Give moderate (15-pound) pressure with both thumbs for three seconds. Pause.

2 Move down approximately two finger-widths with both thumbs. Repeat the pressures. Pause.

3 Continue down at two finger-width intervals until you are on a line with the base of the spine.

4 Move back to the shoulders and place each of your thumbs another inch further out from the spine. Follow the previous sequence giving moderate (15-pound) pressure down to a point on a line with the base of the spine.

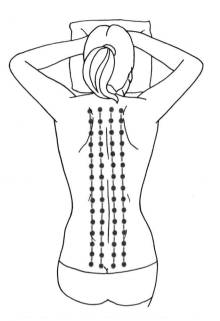

SHOULDER BLADES AND BUTTOCKS

Shoulder Blades

Still straddling your partner, either standing, kneeling or sitting back lightly on your lower legs, probe the right shoulder blade until you locate the deeply recessed area in the center. This, another "Yipe" point, for some strange reason is named "Celestial Ancestor." It is an important point in treating pain from bursitis, tennis elbow, stiff neck and sore shoulder.

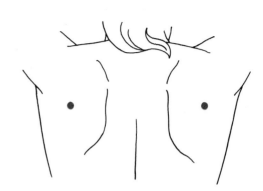

1 Place your thumbs side by side at the recessed center of the blade. Give deep (20-pound) pressure for three seconds. Pause.

2 Repeat the pressure.

3 Give the same pressures with your thumbs side by side at the recessed center point of the left shoulder blade.

Buttocks

You have to shift your position to work on the buttock points. Kneel facing your partner's right hip, lean toward it and locate the point right above the fattest part of the buttock in a direct line with the shoulder blades. This is a "Yipe" point.

1 Keeping your arms straight, place your thumbs side by side in the center of the recess and give deep (20-pound) pressure for three seconds. Pause.

2 Repeat the pressure.

3 Move to your partner's left side, kneel, and give the same deep pressure to the center of the left buttock.

Before you move on to the legs and feet both you and your partner should rest for a few moments. Your thumbs and fingers probably feel stiff or slightly sore. This is to be expected the first few times you give shiatzu. Flex your fingers and hands, take some deep breaths through your nose and exhale slowly through your teeth. Then back to shiatzu.

LEGS AND FEET

The sequences which follow take you down the right leg to the sole of the foot. When you finish the foot you then move to your partner's left and repeat the same sequences.

Upper Leg

Assume a kneeling position outside your partner's right knee. The points on the back of the thigh muscle are on a line down the center of the muscle, which begins where the buttock meets the top of the leg and traces down to a point just above the inside of the knee. The point on this line midway between the buttock and the knee is the most important and sensitive point on the upper leg. It is called the "Great Gate."

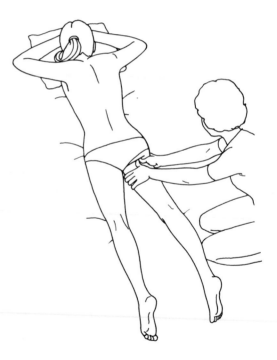

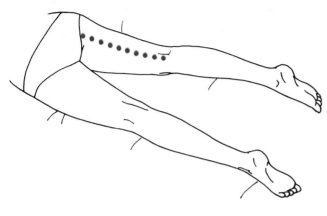

1   Place your thumbs side by side at the top point just under the buttock. Give deep (20-pound) pressure for three seconds. Pause.

2   Move your thumbs two finger-widths down toward the knee. Repeat the deep pressure. Pause.

3   Continue down at two finger-width intervals to the knee. The final point is just above the back of the knee.

Outside of the Thigh

The outside thigh points are on a line which begins at the side of the hip below the hipbone and goes down the center of the side of the thigh. Start below the hip and work down to the side of the knee.

1   Use both thumbs side by side and give deep (20-pound) pressure for three seconds. Pause.

2   Move your thumbs toward the knee two finger-widths. Repeat the pressure. Pause.

3   Continue along the line bisecting the side of the muscle at consistent intervals to the knee.

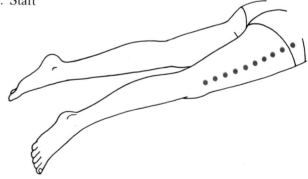

Inside of the Thigh

Move to your partner's left side and reach across to give shiatzu to the inside of the right thigh. The points are on a line that begins at the top of the inside of the leg and bisects the inside of the thigh muscle. It ends at the inside of the knee.

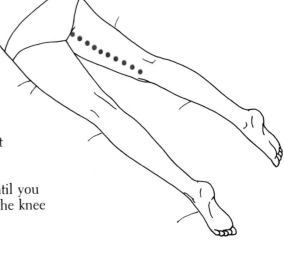

1   Place your thumbs side by side and give deep (20-pound) pressure at the top point for three seconds. Pause.

2   Move along the muscle two finger-widths toward the knee. Repeat the pressure. Pause.

3   Repeat the pressure at two finger-width intervals along the line until you reach the knee. The final point is in the recess midway between the knee bone and the tendons at the back of the knee.

The Calf Muscle

You give shiatzu to the calf muscle in much the same manner as you did to the upper leg. Take a position below your partner's right foot. Reach forward to the top of the calf just below the inside of the knee. This point, called the "Meeting of Yang," is one of the most important points on the body. When the muscles of the leg are tight, this point becomes extremely tense and tender. Shiatzu here releases tension. Place both thumbs side by side at the top of the line which runs down to the center of the back of the ankle.

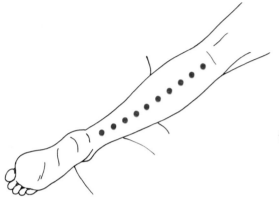

1 Apply deep (20-pound) pressure with thumbs side by side to the point at the top of the muscle. Hold for three seconds. Pause.

2 Move down the center of the muscle two finger-widths and repeat the pressure. Pause.

3 Continue down the muscle at two finger-width intervals. The final pressure point is where the muscle flattens out at the top of the ankle.

Ankle

You must reposition yourself. Kneel alongside your partner's right knee, facing the ankle. Bend forward and place your right thumb on the inside of the ankle at the deepest recess between the anklebone and the back of the ankle (the Achilles tendon). Place your left thumb on the corresponding point at the outside of the ankle.

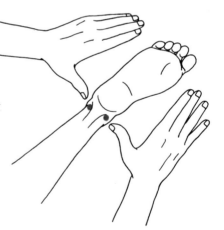

1 Give moderate (15-pound) pressure with both thumbs for three seconds. Pause.

2 Repeat the pressure for three seconds.

Sole

Move back to a position below your partner's right foot. There are four points on the sole which should receive pressure. The first three are on a line which bisects the foot, one of which is appropriately called the "Fountain of Energy." These points are effective in helping to alleviate fatigue and improving circulation throughout the entire body. The fourth point is called the "Valley of the Sole." It is high in and to the back of the arch, above and slightly forward of the first point.

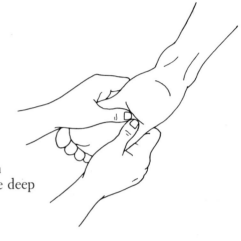

1   Grip the foot with both hands and place both thumbs side by side just in front of the heel pad. Wrap your fingers around the top of the foot. Give deep (20-pound) pressure for three seconds. Pause.

2   Move down the line to the center (the narrowest part) of the foot. Give deep (20-pound) pressure for three seconds. Pause.

3   The third point is just behind the ball of the foot. Give deep (20-pound) pressure for three seconds. Pause.

4   Shift your hands and place both thumbs side by side on the point high in the arch. Give deep pressure for three seconds.
You are now ready to move to your partner's left leg. Follow the sequences and positions described, starting on page 102, and move down from the thigh to the sole of the foot. When you finish the left leg, it is time for

your partner to turn over and rest on her back. And it will be time for you to relax again for a few moments. Take some deep breaths and stretch and flex your fingers and hands. You will then be ready to begin the second half of partner-shiatzu.

NECK, ARMS, AND HANDS

Neck

Kneel to the right of your partner's upper body. You should be able to reach the neck comfortably without stretching your arms. Although specific points are shown in the illustration, you need to use them only as a general guide. The idea is to cover the neck area thoroughly. Just cover the general area, starting beneath the jaw and working down to the base of the neck. Use the index and middle fingers of both hands, alternating your right and left hands.

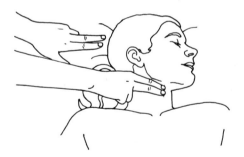

1 Place the index and middle fingers of your right hand under the jaw beside the top of the windpipe. Give light (10-pound) pressure at the top of a line made by the side of the windpipe and the muscle. Be careful not to press directly on the windpipe, but into the muscle. Hold for two seconds. Pause.

2 Place the index and middle fingers of your left hand just below the point you have just pressed with your right hand. Repeat the light pressure.

3 Continue to move straight down alongside the windpipe, alternating your hands to give light pressure, until you reach the base of the neck. In Oriental medicine this is known as the "Fountain of Beauty and Youth."

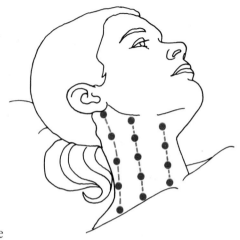

4 Bring your hands back up to the top of the neck underneath the jaw. Repeat the pressures, alternating your hands, along a descending line to the base of the neck.

5 Continue the pressures from the top of the neck to the base until you have covered the front and side of the neck. Hold each pressure for three seconds.

6 Move over to your partner's left side and repeat the sequences on the left of the neck.

Upper Arm

Kneel approximately a foot away from your partner's right hip. Reach forward and with your thumbs side by side place them on the outside of the arm muscle at a point an inch or so below the top of the shoulder. Wrap the fingers of both hands lightly around the arm.

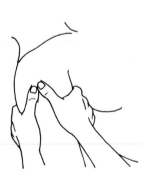

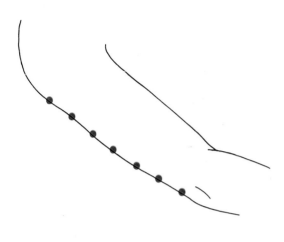

1 Give deep (20-pound) pressure with the thumbs for three seconds. Pause.

2 Slide your thumbs down two finger-widths on a line which leads from the center of the shoulder joint to the side of the elbow. Repeat the pressure. Pause.

3 Repeat the pressures at distances of two finger-widths down to the elbow.

Lower Arm

The lower arm points are on a line which begins at the outside center of the elbow, travels down the center of the forearm, and ends at the midpoint of the back of the wrist. Place the thumbs side by side on the outside of the elbow joint and wrap your fingers lightly around the forearm.

1 Give deep (20-pound) pressure for three seconds at the point on the side of the elbow. Pause.

2 Apply pressure at two finger-width intervals for three seconds each, down the line. The final point is at the center of the back of the wrist.

Back of the Hand

Significant shiatzu points are located in the "ditches" between the tendons which run from the wrist to the base knuckles of each of the fingers. Have your partner spread the fingers of her right hand.

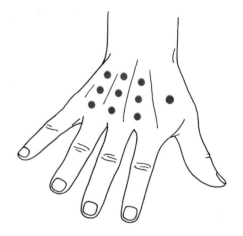

1 Place your right thumb on the back of your partner's hand on the mound of muscle above the hollow where her thumb joins her hand. Place your right index finger directly underneath on the palm.

2 Squeeze with deep (20-pound) pressure for three seconds. This is a "Yipe" point, and known in Oriental medicine as the "Valley." Pause.

3 Move your thumb to the ditch between your partner's index and middle fingers midway between the wrist and base knuckle. Move your index finger directly underneath on the palm.

4 Give moderate (15-pound) pressure by squeezing for three seconds. Pause.

5 Moving down the ditch, repeat the pressure at two more points, ending between the knuckles.

6 Repeat the entire sequence in the ditches between the tendons of the middle and third fingers, and then again in the ditches between the third and little finger.

Fingers

In Oriental medicine it is believed that the thumb is related to the function of the lungs; the index finger is related to the large intestine; the middle finger, the heart; the third finger, the respiratory, digestive and circulatory systems; the little finger, the heart. I believe that shiatzu of the fingers is important in keeping the organs in a healthy condition. The thumb and each of the fingers should receive pressure at the top, bottom, and sides of each of the individual finger bones.

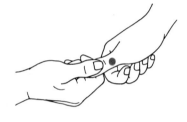

1 Begin with your partner's right thumb. Place your thumb at the midpoint between the base knuckle and the joint. Place your index finger on the underside directly opposite your thumb. Give moderate (15-pound) pressure for three seconds.

2 Move toward the end of the thumb. Place your thumb on the base of your partner's thumbnail. Your index finger should be directly underneath. Give moderate squeezing pressure for three seconds.

3 Move back toward the base knuckle and at the midpoint of the bone give moderate squeezing pressure on both sides of the thumb simultaneously. Pause.

4 Repeat the pressure at the sides of the thumbnail.

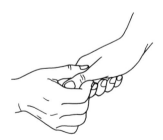

5 Give pressure to each of your partner's fingers in the same manner. Follow along the top and underside of the finger, then along the sides. Then move on to the next finger.

Inside of the Upper Arm

Kneel a few feet away from your partner's midsection so that you can comfortably work on the right upper arm. Have your partner extend her arm away from the side of her body. Roll it slightly so that you are looking down at the inside of the arm. The line to follow here begins deep in the center of the armpit, runs alongside the muscle where it meets the inside of the upper arm bone, and ends at the inside center of the elbow. The point at the center of the armpit is called "Depth of the Pond," for it is from here that blood moves out to the entire arm.

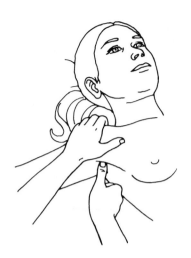

1 Grasp the corner of your partner's right shoulder with your left hand. Place your right thumb deep in the armpit.

2 Give deep (20-pound) pressure for two seconds. Pause. This is a "Yipe" point and if you are on the mark your partner will react loudly.

3 Placate your partner and then move both your thumbs down to the top of the inside of the major arm muscle. With your fingers wrapped lightly around the arm give deep (20-pound) pressure with your thumbs side by side. Hold for three seconds. Pause.

4 Move toward the elbow along the muscle/bone line at intervals of two finger-widths. Give deep pressure for three seconds. Pause.

5 Continue applying the side-by-side thumb pressure at two finger-width intervals until you reach the inside of the elbow.

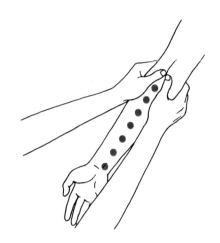

Inside of the Lower Arm

The points on the lower arm run on a line from the center of the elbow directly down the center of the inside of the arm to the center of the wrist.

1 Place your thumbs side by side at the inside center of the elbow. Wrap your fingers lightly around the joint.

2 Give deep (20-pound) pressure with both thumbs deep in the center of the elbow. This is another "Yipe" point.

3 Move two finger-widths down the line bisecting the inside of the forearm. Give deep pressure for three seconds. Pause.

4 Continue down this line at two finger-width intervals, giving three-second deep pressure until you reach the wrist. The inside center of the wrist is the final point.

Palm

Three points on the palm of each hand should receive pressure. The first is at the center of the muscle that forms the heel of the hand, the second is just beyond the muscle where it dips down into the palm. The third, called the "Temple of Fatigue," is effective in helping to alleviate fatigue and improve circulation throughout the entire body. It is in the direct center of the palm.

1 Hold your partner's hand, palm up, by placing the little finger of your right hand between your partner's little finger and third finger. Place the little finger of your left hand between your partner's index finger and thumb.

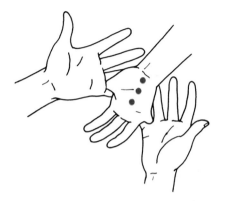

2 Using both of your thumbs side by side, give deep (20-pound) pressure at the center of the heel muscle for three seconds. Pause.

3 Repeat the pressure on each of the remaining palm joints for three seconds.

You should now move to your partner's left and work on the left arm. Repeat the sequences for the upper arm, lower arm, hands, fingers, inside of the upper arm, inside of the lower arm and palm. When you finish you will probably once again feel a need for a momentary rest. This is a good place to do it.

LEGS, FEET AND TOES

Upper Leg

Kneel alongside your partner's right lower leg. Face toward the hip. The shiatzu points on the front of the upper leg run down the center of the leg muscle from the front of the hip joint down to a point just above the center of the knee.

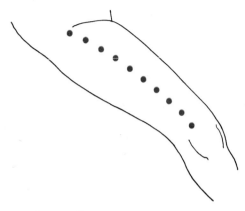

1 Place both thumbs at the top center of the leg. Wrap your fingers lightly around the muscle. Give deep (20-pound) pressure for three seconds. Pause.

2 Move your thumbs two finger-widths toward the knee. Give deep pressure for three seconds. Pause.

3 Continue to the point just above the knee, giving deep pressure at two finger-width intervals.

Lower Leg

Kneel approximately a foot away from the side of your partner's right lower leg. Face directly toward the leg, lean forward and place both thumbs side by side on the outside of the shin at the muscle line just below the kneecap. Extend your fingers over the leg and grip the other side of the shinbone so that it is being squeezed between thumb and fingers. Your fingers are gripping a point called "Walking Three Miles." In ancient times people used to stop by roadside inns after a lengthy walk to receive moxibustion (a treatment in which a small quantity of an herb called moxa was burned on the skin, acting as a counterirritant) or acupuncture on this point to eliminate leg fatigue and cramps.

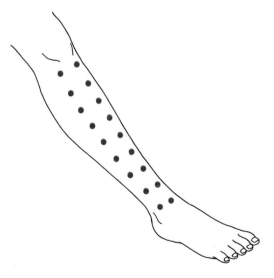

1 Begin at the top of the bone and give deep (20-pound) pressure with fingers and thumbs of both hands in a squeezing motion. Pause.

2 Move three finger-widths down toward the ankle. Repeat the thumb and finger pressure for three seconds. Pause.

3 Continue this pressure down the lower leg until you reach the ankle. The final point is at the top of the instep.

Foot

Take a position facing your partner's feet as you kneel alongside the right knee. The points on the feet are similar to those on the hands. They are located in the "ditches" between the tendons that lead to the toes. Start on the top of the right foot.

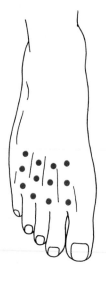

1 Place your thumbs side by side in the small ditch approximately two inches above the base of the large toe and the first toe. Grip with your thumbs on top of the foot and your index fingers on the sole.

2 Give moderate (15-pound) pressure for three seconds. Pause.

3 Move forward halfway to the toes. Give moderate pressure for three seconds. Pause.

4 The third point is right at the end of the ditch. Give moderate pressure for three seconds. Pause.

5 Repeat the sequence in the ditch between each of the tendons leading to the toes.

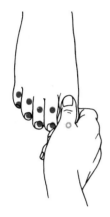

Toes

Begin with the big toe. Again, as with the fingers, there are points midway between the joints on the top, bottom and sides of each small bone.

1 Place your right thumb on top of the first bone in the big toe and your index finger directly underneath and opposite. Give moderate (15-pound) squeezing pressure for three seconds. Pause.

2 Place your thumb at the base of the toenail and your index finger directly opposite underneath the toe. Give moderate squeezing pressure for three seconds. Pause.

3 Move back to the first bone of the big toe. Give pressure on both sides of the midpoint of the toe by squeezing. Hold for three seconds. Pause. Then repeat the pressure at the sides of the second bone.

4 Give pressure to each of the toes in the same sequence. Follow along the top and underside of each small bone, then along the sides.

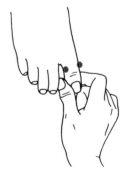

You should now move to your partner's left and repeat the sequences for the upper leg, lower leg, feet and toes.

You are now nearly finished with the shiatzu sequences. Your partner should be feeling extremely relaxed, and it would be unusual for you, as a layperson, to feel anything except the need for another momentary rest. Shake your hands and arms, and then, after some deep breaths, begin the final shiatzu touches on your partner's head and face.

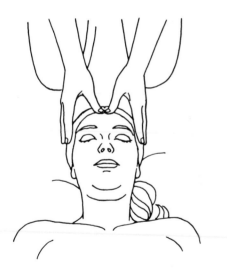

Head and Face

Kneel beyond the top of your partner's head. Measure the distance by leaning forward and extending your arms. You should be able to reach the top of the head without stretching.

Top of the Head

Shiatzu on the top of the head is very effective in relaxing your partner and giving her a feeling of euphoria. The area that concerns you first starts at the hairline and is inside the perimeter of the hair.

1 Place both thumbs side by side at the midpoint of the hairline, at the widow's peak. Give moderate (15-pound) pressure for three seconds. Pause.

2 Move your thumbs back two finger-widths along the line of an imaginary center part in her hair. Give moderate (15-pound) pressure for three seconds. Pause.

3 Continue back to the rear of the crown at intervals of two finger-widths. Give moderate pressure for three seconds at each point.

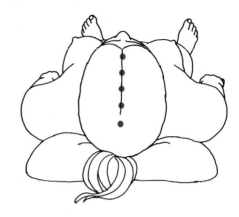

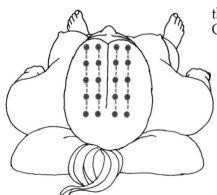

4 Move your hands back to the center of the hairline. Separate them, moving your right thumb a third of the way out to the right side of the head, the left thumb a third of the distance to the left side. Place the thumbs at these points on the hairline. Give moderate (15-pound) pressure for three seconds. Pause.

5 Move your thumbs back toward the rear of the head two finger-widths. Give moderate pressure for three seconds. Pause.

6 Continue giving pressure at two finger-width intervals until you reach the rear of the crown.

7 Come back again to the hairline and move your thumbs an equal distance out to the sides of the head. Give moderate pressure for three seconds at two finger-width intervals until you again reach the rear of the crown.

Forehead

These shiatzu points are located along five vertical lines on the forehead. The first line runs straight down from the widow's peak. The next pair of lines runs down to the midpoint of the eyebrows. The last pair of lines runs down to the outside of the eyebrows.

1 Still kneeling beyond your partner's head, lean forward and place your thumbs side by side at the midpoint of the hairline.

2 Give moderate (15-pound) pressure for three seconds. Pause.

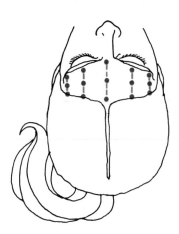

3 Move your thumbs down two finger-widths. Give moderate pressure for three seconds. Pause.

4 Continue down to the midpoint between the eyebrows.

5 Move back to the hairline, separate your thumbs and place the right thumb at the hairline point above the center of the right eyebrow and the left thumb at the point above the left eyebrow. Give moderate pressure for three seconds. Pause.

6 Continue down the lines with moderate pressure. The final point on these lines is just above the center of the eyebrows.

7 Starting at the points above the outside edges of the eyebrows, give pressure along the lines down to and including the final points at the outside edge of each eyebrow.

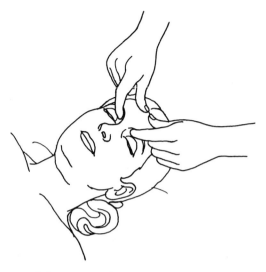

Eyes

The points surrounding the eyes are on the inside edge of the eye sockets. Use the index fingers of both hands and do points on the right and left eyes simultaneously. If your partner is wearing contact lenses, they should be removed.

1 Place your index fingers on the upper ridges of the eye sockets, as close to the nose as possible.

2 Give light (10-pound) pressure directly on the inner edge of the socket bones for three seconds. Pause.

3 Move your fingers toward the outside of the eyes approximately one finger-width. Repeat the light pressures for three seconds. Keep the bulbs of your fingers directly on the inner edge of the socket bones. Pause.

4 Continue the pressures at consistent intervals until you have covered the points at the outside of the sockets.

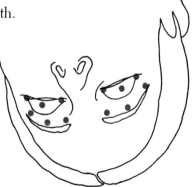

5 Lean forward and place the index and middle fingers of each hand on your partner's closed eyelids. Give gentle (2- to 3-pound) pressure with the flats of your fingers. Hold for three seconds.
Change position to work on the lower ridge of the eye sockets. Kneel close to your partner's midsection.

1 Give light (10-pound) pressure directly on the inner edge of the bones for three seconds. Pause.

2 Move your fingers out along the lower edge of the sockets one finger-width. Repeat the light pressures for three seconds. Pause.

3 Continue the pressures at one finger-width intervals to the outside edge of the sockets.

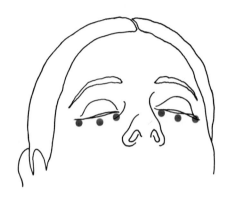

Cheeks

Return to your position above your partner's head. You give pressure to the points of the cheekbones by placing the tip of your third finger on top of the nail of your index finger. Do this with both your right and left hands.

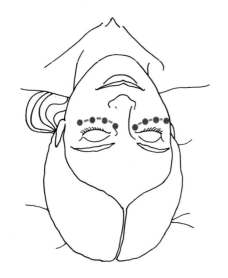

1 Give moderate (15-pound) pressure at the outside edge of the nose, slightly below the bridge of the nose. Do both the right and left sides simultaneously. Hold for three seconds. Pause.

2 Move your fingers out one finger-width onto the cheekbones, toward the sides of the face. Give moderate (15-pound) pressure for three seconds. Pause.

3 Move another finger-width out on the cheekbones. Give moderate pressure for three seconds. Pause.

4 Move one more finger-width out on the cheekbones. Hold the moderate pressure for three seconds.

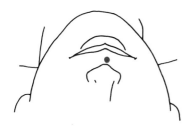

Mouth and Chin

There are four points near the mouth. The first is midway between the bottom of the nose and the upper lip. The second and third (a pair) are on the cheeks three finger-widths out from the corners of the mouth. The fourth is in the recess of the chin, midway between the lower lip and the tip of the chin.

1 Use your right thumb. Give moderate (15-pound) pressure on the point between the nose and the upper lip.

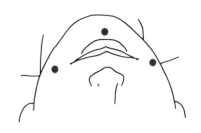

2   Hold for three seconds. Pause.

3   Using both thumbs simultaneously give moderate (15-pound) pressure at the points beyond the corners of the mouth. Hold for three seconds. Pause.

4   Place your thumb on the point midway between the lower lip and the tip of the chin. Give moderate pressure for three seconds.

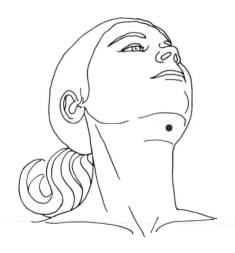

Under Chin

Move to your partner's right side and kneel by her waist. The point under the chin is located behind the front of the lower jawbone. Reach under the chin, two finger-widths in from the tip. Place the bulb of your second finger in the recess behind the bone.

1   Give moderate (15-pound) pressure for three seconds. Pause.

2   Repeat the pressure.

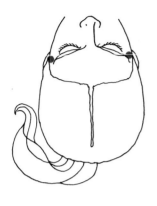

Temples

Move back to above your partner's head. The final points are on the right and left temples. Do both sides simultaneously.

1 Use both hands. Place the tips of your middle fingers on top of the index fingers. Locate the slight recesses on the sides of the temples. Give moderate (15-pound) pressure to both temples.

2 Hold the pressure for three seconds. Pause.

3 Repeat the pressure.

Final Exercises

The shiatzu pressure sequences are now completed. All that remains are the final relaxing movements.

1 Have your partner extend her arms out on the floor above her head.

2 Grip her hands and gently pull, stretching her arms as much as possible.

3 Have your partner stretch her legs and toes and take a deep breath through her nose.

4 Have her exhale slowly through her mouth. At the same time instruct her to relax her legs and toes, and release your grip from her hands.

Your partner should rest for at least five minutes before getting up. When she does rise she may experience momentary dizziness or light-headedness. But within a few seconds she should have her bearings. She should feel a deep sense of satisfaction and fulfillment and a warm, tingling sensation from head to foot.

In the days following full-body partner-shiatzu, most people experience one of two aftereffect patterns. Often people feel completely relaxed, peaceful, and sleepy immediately after shiatzu. They will sleep soundly that night. The next day they feel relaxed but slightly tired. Then, on the second day, they experience a strong sense of physical and emotional well-being. They are full of energy and feel they have the capacity to work to the peak of their ability. This condition, depending upon the individual, usually lasts from two to five days.

The second pattern is one of an immediate surge of energy after partner-shiatzu. These people feel relaxed, but energetic and elated, almost euphoric—some people compare it to feeling high. This condition lasts for several hours immediately after partner-shiatzu. Then they feel a sudden heavy fatigue, yet they sleep only fitfully the first night. The following day they feel relaxed and somewhat tired. They sleep deeply the second night and awaken to a sense of well-being, full of physical and mental energy. This condition—also depending on the individual—lasts from two to five days.

Because of the intensely individual reactions to receiving full-body partner-shiatzu, I feel that it is ideally given and received in the late afternoon or early evening, and for maximum long-range results it should be repeated at five- to seven-day intervals. Consistency is important in giving and gaining the true benefits of shiatzu: health, vitality and serenity.

Part II

Shiatzu as a Remedy for Disorders

One of the most dramatic and rewarding experiences shiatzu can provide is a good night's sleep.

I have often given shiatzu to people with specific sleeping problems. I once gave shiatzu to a sixty-two-year-old man who had suffered from insomnia off and on for forty years. He couldn't get to sleep without sleeping pills. An internationally known authority on painting, he was active in many cultural organizations and had boundless energy coupled with a highly explosive and oversensitive disposition.

From his first experience with shiatzu his sleep improved and he felt an enormous sense of relaxation. With each successive experience sleep came easier until, after two months of weekly treatments, he stopped taking pills and was able to fall asleep naturally.

In my experience of giving shiatzu to people with sleeping problems I have found that, without exception, their neck muscles are extremely tense. So in all applications of shiatzu for insomnia I pay particular attention to the muscles of the neck. In addition, I concentrate on the muscles of the shoulders and the abdomen.

If you or your partner has difficulty getting to sleep, a nightly application of shiatzu just before bedtime will bring some improvement immediately. Continue these nightly exercises until the problem disappears. The length of time required to overcome recurring insomnia will vary with such factors as age, physical condition, the length of time the condition has existed, and the kind of life you lead. But once the problem disappears, you can keep it from returning with two applications a week. A hot bath just before shiatzu will relax the muscles and makes shiatzu for insomnia even more effective.

Chapter 7

Insomnia

SELF-SHIATZU FOR INSOMNIA

Top of the Head

Begin the self-shiatzu sequence while you are sitting up on the side of your bed. Place the index and middle fingers of both hands side by side on the center of the top of your crown.

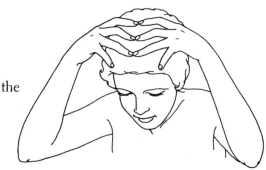

1 Give deep (20-pound) pressure for three seconds. Pause.

2 Repeat the pressure. Pause.

3 Repeat the pressure once more.

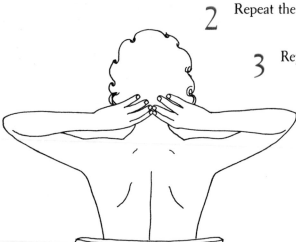

Base of the Skull

Reach both hands behind your head and place the index and middle fingers of both hands in the slight indentation in the center of the top of the neck, just below the base of the skull.

1   Give deep (20-pound) pressure for three seconds. Pause.

2   Repeat the pressure. Pause.

3   Repeat the pressure again. Pause.

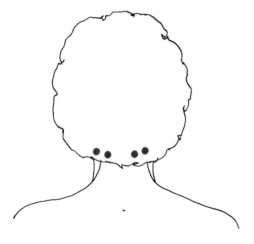

4   Move your left hand out along the base of the skull two finger-widths to the left and the right hand two finger-widths to the right. Give deep (20-pound) pressure with the index and middle fingers of both hands simultaneously. Pause.

5   Repeat the pressure twice more, as above.

6   Move each hand out along the base of the skull two more finger-widths. Give deep (20-pound) pressure with the index and middle fingers of both hands simultaneously. Pause.

7   Repeat the pressure twice more.

Neck Muscles

Place the index and middle fingers of your left hand at the top of the large muscle which runs down the left side of the back of the neck from the base of the skull to the shoulder line. Place the index and middle fingers of your right hand at the corresponding point on the right side of the back of the neck.

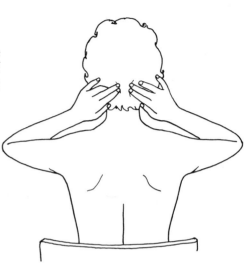

1 Give deep (20-pound) pressure on both points simultaneously for three seconds. Pause.

2 Repeat the pressure. Pause.

3 Repeat the pressure again. Pause.

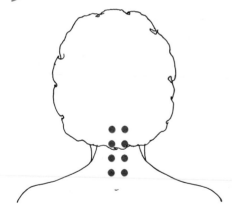

4 Move down the muscle lines two finger-widths, with your fingers centered on the muscle bands. Give deep (20-pound) pressure for three seconds. Pause.

5 Repeat the deep pressure two more times.

6 Continue down the neck muscles at two finger-width intervals, giving deep (20-pound) pressure for three seconds three times at each point. Pause for a second after each pressure. The final points are at the base of the muscles, at the shoulder line.

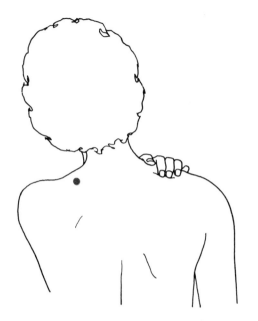

Shoulders

Find the point on top of your right shoulder with the index and middle fingers of your left hand. The point is halfway between the base of the neck and the edge of your shoulder. Probe slightly to the rear of the shoulder muscle with your fingers. When you are on the most tender spot you have found the point.

1 Give deep (20-pound) pressure with both fingers for three seconds. Pause.

2 Repeat the pressure. Pause.

3 Repeat the pressure again. Pause.

4 Repeat the sequence on the center point of your left shoulder, using the index and middle fingers of your right hand.

Upper Back

This sequence requires some stretching, but don't worry if you can't seem to reach the points at first; the longer you maintain the nightly practice of shiatzu for insomnia, the easier this sequence will become.

Reach your left hand over your right shoulder as far down the right side of your spine as your arm will stretch. Use your index, middle and third fingers, with the third finger next to the spine.

1   Give deep (20-pound) pressure with all three fingers simultaneously for three seconds. Pause.

2   Repeat the deep pressure. Pause.

3   Repeat the pressure again. Pause.

4   Move about two finger-widths up the back toward your shoulders, keeping your three fingers between the spine and the shoulder blade. Give deep (20-pound) pressure for three seconds. Pause.

5   Repeat the pressure twice more. Pause.

6   Move two finger-widths further up the back and give deep (20-pound) pressure three times for three seconds each, as before.

7   Move two finger-widths further up the back. By now you should be at the shoulder line. Repeat the three deep pressures.

8   Now reach your right hand back over your left shoulder as far as you can and repeat the sequence on the left side of your spine.

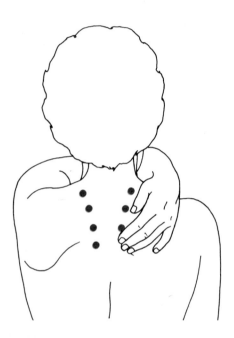

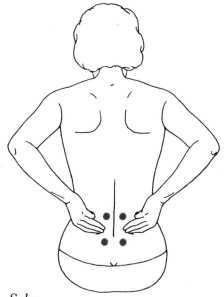

Lower Back

Place your hands on your lower back with the index, middle and third fingers of both hands on the sides of the spine at the waistline. The third finger of each hand should be about two finger-widths from the spine.

1 Give moderate (15-pound) pressure with the index, middle and third fingers of both hands simultaneously for three seconds. Pause.

2 Repeat the pressure. Pause.

3 Move both hands about two finger-widths down your back and repeat the moderate pressure. Pause. Repeat the pressure again. Pause.

4 Move your hands about two finger-widths further down the back. You should be near the top of your buttocks. Give moderate (15-pound) pressure with both hands simultaneously, pause, and repeat the pressure.

Soles

Rest your right leg on your left knee. Four points on the sole of each foot receive pressure. The first three are on a line which bisects the foot from the center of the heel through the middle toe. The fourth is high in the arch, toward the rear, near the corner of the heel.

1 Wrap your hands around your foot and place both thumbs side by side just in front of your heel pad. Give deep (20-pound) pressure for three seconds. Pause.

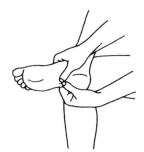

2 Move down the center line to the narrowest part of the foot and repeat the pressure. Pause.

3 Move down the center line to the point just behind the ball of the foot. Repeat the deep (20-pound) pressure. Pause.

4 Now place your thumbs side by side on the point high in the arch. Give deep pressure for three seconds. Pause.

5 Go back and repeat the sequence two more times.

6 Lift your left leg up onto your right knee and perform the sequence three times on your left foot.

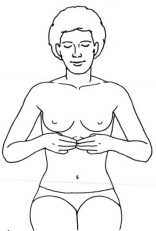

Abdomen

Although all the sequences that follow are shown being done while you are seated, you may also do them lying down.

The points on the abdomen run vertically down five lines along the abdomen, between the bottom of the rib cage and the groin. The first line runs down the center of the abdomen. Then a pair of lines runs down either side of the center line. Finally, there is a pair of lines still further out from the center. After going down the center line, press the points on the right side before proceeding to those on the left.

1 Place the index, middle and third fingers of both hands side by side just below the breastbone in the center of the rib cage. Give moderate (15-pound) pressure for three seconds. Pause.

2 Move down the center line two finger-widths and repeat the moderate pressure. Pause.

3 Continue down the center line at two finger-width intervals, giving moderate pressure for three seconds at each point, until you reach the groin.

4 Move your hands over four finger-widths to the right of the center line. Place the index, middle and third fingers of both hands just below the bottom rib. Give moderate (15-pound) pressure for three seconds. Pause.

5 Proceed down the line at two finger-width intervals, as above, giving moderate pressure at each point for three seconds, until you reach the base of the trunk.

6 Move your hands over four finger-widths further to the right. Place the index, middle and third fingers directly below the bottom rib. Give moderate (15-pound) pressure for three seconds. Pause. Continue down in the same manner at two finger-width intervals to the fold at the top of the leg.

7 Now move over to your left side, four finger-widths out from the center line, and repeat the same series of pressures at two finger-width intervals until you reach the base of the trunk.

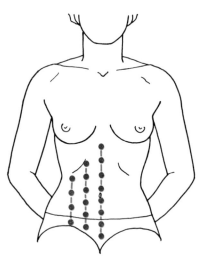

8 Now move over to the line four finger-widths further to the left and repeat the sequence until you reach the fold at the top of the leg.

9 Finally, place both your palms on your abdomen. Give light (10-pound), even pressure with both palms simultaneously. Move your palms so that you cover your abdomen with gentle pressure. Concentrate on areas that feel most tense until they relax.

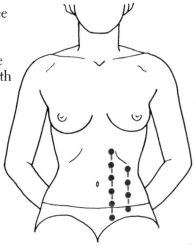

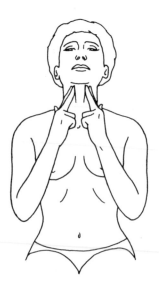

Front and Sides of the Neck

Use the index and middle fingers of both hands to do the points on the neck. The specific points shown in the illustration are only for general guidance. The idea is to cover the area shown. Do corresponding points on both right and left sides at the same time.

1 Place the index and middle fingers of the right hand under your jaw at the right side of the top of your windpipe, and the same fingers of the left hand at the same point on the left side. Give light (10-pound) pressure at these points for two seconds, pressing down into the muscle, not the windpipe. Pause.

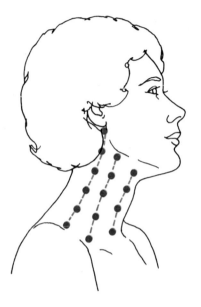

2 Move both hands down the line slightly and continue to give light pressure for two seconds at points along the line down to the base of the neck.

3 Return to the top of the neck underneath the jaw, slightly further along the jawline toward the sides of the neck. Repeat the pressures on both sides of the neck along a descending line to the base.

4 Continue this procedure, lightly pressing from the top of the neck to the base, starting each time further out to the side of the neck, until you have covered the front and sides of the neck.

Temples

There are two points on each side of the head. Do corresponding points on both sides simultaneously, with the middle finger of each hand on top of the nail of the index finger.

1 Place your fingers on the first pair of points in the recesses about two finger-widths beyond the outside corners of your eyes and a little above them.

2 Give moderate (15-pound) pressure for three seconds. Pause.

3 Move your hands up to the second pair of points, one finger-width up, and two back, and repeat the pressure.

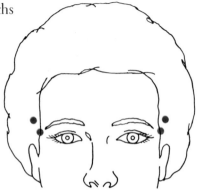

Palms

There are four points on the palm that receive pressure. The first three are on a line which runs from the center of the wrist to the base of the middle finger. The fourth is on the heel of the thumb.

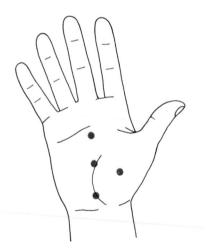

1 Place your left thumb in the center of the fleshy area at the base of the right palm. Wrap your fingers around the back of your hand. Give deep (20-pound) pressure for three seconds. Pause.

2 Move down the line to the center of your right palm and repeat the deep pressure for three seconds. Pause.

3 Place your left thumb on the fleshy pad at the base of your right middle finger and repeat the deep pressure. Pause.

4 Move over to the point on the heel of the thumb and give deep (20-pound) pressure.

5 Go back and repeat the entire sequence once more on the right hand.

6 Repeat the entire sequence twice on the left hand.

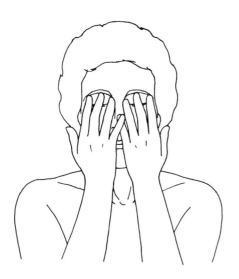

Eyes

The points surrounding the eyes are on the inside edges of the eye sockets. Use the index, middle and third fingers of the left hand for the points on the left eye, and the index, middle and third fingers of the right hand for the points on the right eye. If you are wearing contact lenses, remove them.

1 Spread your fingers slightly and place the bulbs on the inside of the upper ridges of the sockets. The third finger of each hand should be as close to the nose as possible. Press the tips of your fingers upward against the inner edges of the sockets, giving light (10-pound) pressure for three seconds. Pause.

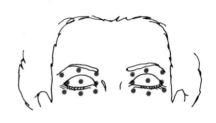

2 Bring the fingers down slightly, resting the bulbs on your closed eyelids. Press gently (2 to 3 pounds) for three seconds. Pause.

3 Arch your fingers slightly and press against the inner edge of the lower ridges of the eye sockets. Use light (10-pound) pressure for three seconds.

4 Go back and repeat the entire sequence one more time.

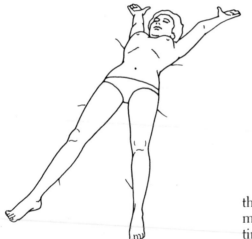

Final Exercises

Lie down on your back, stretch your arms, legs and toes and slowly inhale through your nose. Gradually relax your muscles as you exhale through your mouth, making a hissing noise through your front teeth. Repeat this at least six times.

PARTNER-SHIATZU FOR INSOMNIA

The partner-shiatzu for insomnia exercises are designed to be done comfortably on a bed. Your partner should be lying on his stomach for the first sequences. Since you won't have enough room on your bed to position yourself above the top of your partner's head, sit astride with your weight on your lower legs.

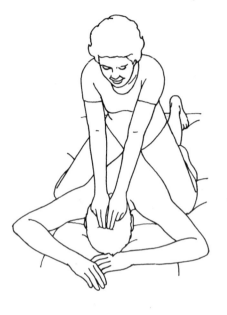

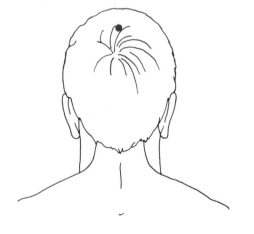

Back of the Crown

The first point is on the center of the top of the crown.

1 Place the index and middle fingers of both hands on this point. Give deep (20-pound) pressure for three seconds. Pause.

2 Repeat the deep pressure. Pause.

3 Repeat the pressure once more.

Central Shoulder Points

Extend your right arm, place your right index and middle fingers at the center of your partner's right shoulder.

1 Give deep (20-pound) pressure for three seconds. Pause.

2 Repeat the deep pressure for three seconds. Pause.

3 Repeat the pressure once more. Pause.

4 Reverse the position of your hands, placing your left on the center rear shoulder point on your partner's left shoulder. Give deep (20-pound) pressure for three seconds. Pause.

5 Repeat the deep pressure two more times.

Base of the Skull

Place your left thumb on top of your right thumb in the slight indentation in the center of the top of the neck, just below the base of the skull.

1 Give deep (20-pound) pressure with both thumbs for three seconds. Pause.

2   Repeat the pressure. Pause.

3   Repeat the pressure again. Pause.

4   Move both your thumbs out along the base of the skull two finger-widths to
    your partner's right. Give deep (20-pound) pressure with both thumbs for
three seconds. Pause.

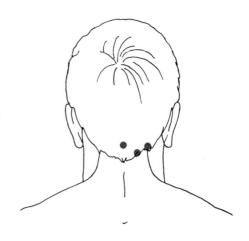

5   Repeat the pressure twice more.

6   Move both your thumbs out along the base of the skull two more finger-widths
    to your partner's right. Give deep (20-pound) pressure for three seconds. Pause.

7   Repeat the pressures two more times.

8   Now move out along the base of the skull to your partner's left, first two, then
    four finger-widths from the center of the neck. Repeat the sequences of three
deep (20-pound) pressures for three seconds at each point. Pause for a second after
each pressure.

Neck Muscles

Move your hands apart. Use the thumb of each hand and place at the top of the major muscles which run down the outside back of the neck from the base of the skull to the shoulders. Place your left thumb at the top of the left muscle where it meets the skull and place your right thumb at the corresponding point at the top of the right muscle.

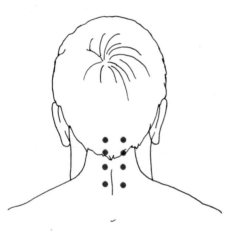

1 Give deep (20-pound) pressure on both points simultaneously for three seconds. Pause.

2 Repeat the pressure. Pause.

3 Repeat the pressure again. Pause.

4 Move down the muscle lines two finger-widths. Center your thumbs on the muscle bands. Give deep (20-pound) pressure for three seconds. Pause.

5 Repeat the deep pressure two more times.

6 Continue down the neck muscles at two finger-width intervals. Give deep (20-pound) pressure for three seconds three times at each point, pausing for a second after each pressure. The final points are at the base of the muscles, on the shoulder line.

Spine

Still straddling your partner, give shiatzu down the entire length of the spine from the base of the neck to the base of the tailbone. Keep your weight resting on your lower legs —not on your partner. Give pressure with arms extended and the weight of your upper body transmitted down to and through your thumbs.

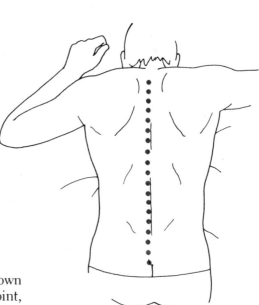

Start at the base of the neck just beneath the bulging bone—the largest you can feel at the shoulder line.

1 Place your right thumb in the recess beneath the bulging bone where it joins the next vertebra. Give moderate (15-pound) pressure for three seconds. Pause.

2 Move down the spine and place your left thumb on the next recessed point. Give moderate (15-pound) pressure for three seconds. Pause.

3 Alternate your thumbs, right, then left, following the recessed points down the spine to the end of the tailbone. Give moderate pressure at each point, then pause and move down.

Right and Left Sides of the Spine

1 Place your left thumb on the shoulder line an inch to the left of the spine and your right thumb an inch to the right of the spine. Give moderate (15-pound) pressure with both thumbs for three seconds. Pause.

2 Move both thumbs down approximately two finger-widths. Repeat the pressure. Pause.

3 Continue moving down at two finger-width intervals all the way to the base of the tailbone. Give moderate (15-pound) pressure with both thumbs for three seconds at each pair of points.

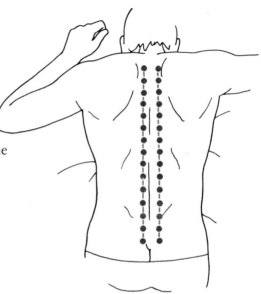

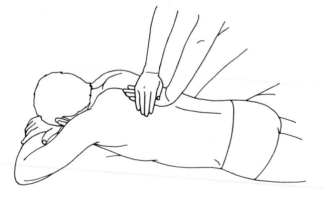

Back

Kneel at your partner's right side. Place your left hand at the top of the spine, pointing toward the head, with the palm flat on the spine. Place your right hand over it at a right angle, pointing toward the left shoulder.

1 Lean straight down upon your palms with the weight of your upper body. Give moderate (15-pound) pressure. Count to ten. Pause.

2 Move down the spine one palm-width and repeat the pressure. Pause.

3 Continue down the spine at one palm-width intervals until you reach the bottom of the spine.

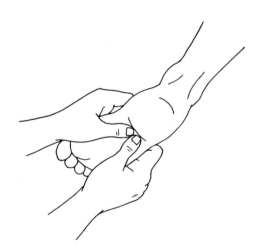

Soles

Move down to a position below your partner's right foot. You may have to get off the bed to do this. You give pressure to four points on the sole of each foot. The first three are on a line which bisects the foot from the center of the heel through the middle toe. The fourth is high in the arch, near the corner of the heel, just forward of the first point.

1 Wrap your fingers around the top of the right foot and place both thumbs side by side just in front of the center of the heel pad. Give deep (20-pound) pressure for three seconds. Pause.

2 Move down the line to the center of the narrowest part of the foot and repeat the pressure. Pause.

3 Move down the line to the point just behind the center of the ball of the foot. Give deep pressure for three seconds. Pause.

4 Shift your hands around slightly and place both thumbs side by side on the point high in the arch. Give deep pressure for three seconds.

5 Go back and repeat the sequence twice more on the right foot.

6 Move over and line yourself up below your partner's left foot. Perform the sequence three times on the left foot.

Abdomen

Have your partner turn over on his back while you kneel at his right side. The points on the abdomen run vertically down five lines between the bottom ribs and the groin. The first line runs down the center of the abdomen from the bottom of the breastbone through the navel to the base of the trunk. The next two lines (a pair) run down the abdomen on either side of the center line. The last two lines (a pair) run down the abdomen still further out to each side. Press corresponding points on both sides simultaneously.

1 Place both thumbs side by side just below the breastbone, in the center of the rib cage. Give moderate (15-pound) pressure for three seconds. Pause.

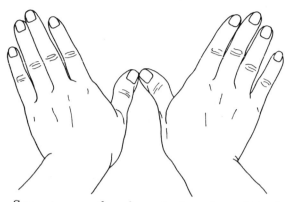

2 Move two finger-widths down the center line and repeat the moderate pressure. Pause.

3 Continue down the center line at two finger-width intervals, giving moderate pressure for three seconds at each point, until you reach the groin.

4 Separate your thumbs and place them directly below the bottom ribs, four finger-widths to either side of the center line. Give moderate (15-pound) pressure for three seconds. Pause.

5 Proceed down these lines at two finger-width intervals, giving moderate pressure at each point for three seconds until you reach the base of the trunk.

6 Now move your thumbs out to the lines eight finger-widths to either side of the center line, just below the bottom ribs. Give moderate (15-pound) pressure for three seconds. Pause.

7 Proceed down these lines at two finger-width intervals, as above, giving moderate pressure at each point for three seconds, until you reach the tops of the legs.

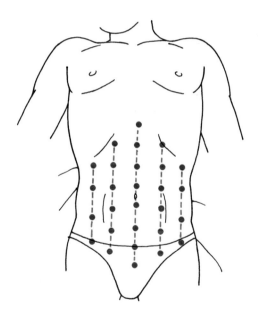

8 Place both hands on your partner's abdomen, palms down. Give light (10-pound) pressure with both palms simultaneously, moving your hands to cover the abdomen with gentle pressure. Concentrate on the areas where the muscles feel most tense until you feel some relaxation.

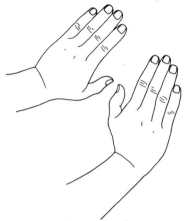

Temples

Again sit lightly astride your partner, resting your weight on your legs. There are two points on each side of the head. The first pair are two finger-widths beyond the outside corners of the eyes. The second are in the shallow recesses of the temples. Give pressure simultaneously to corresponding points on both sides of the head. Place the tips of your middle fingers over the nails of your index fingers and press with both fingers.

1 Place your fingers on the first pair of points and give moderate (15-pound) pressure for three seconds. Pause.

2 Repeat the pressure. Pause.

3 Repeat the pressure again. Pause.

4 Move your hands up to the second pair of points and give moderate (15-pound) pressure for three seconds. Pause.

5 Repeat the pressure two more times.

Eyes

The eye points surround the eyes on the inside edges of the sockets. Use the thumb of each hand and do the points on the right and left eyes simultaneously.

1 Place your thumb on the lower edge of the upper ridges of the eye sockets, as close to the nose as possible.

2 Give light (10-pound) pressure directly on the inner edge of the sockets for three seconds. Pause.

3 Move your thumbs out toward the sides of the face, approximately one finger-width. Repeat the light pressure on the inner edge of the sockets. Hold the pressure for three seconds. Pause.

4 Continue the light (10-pound) pressures at intervals of one finger-width, ending at the points at the outside of the sockets.

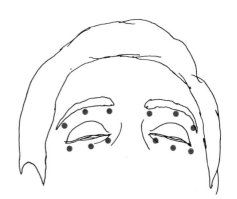

5 Go back to the inside corner of the eyes and repeat the sequence once more.

6 Using your index fingers simultaneously on the right and left eyes, start as close to the nose as possible. Give light (10-pound) pressure directly down on the inner edge of the sockets. Hold the pressure for three seconds. Pause.

7 Move your fingers one finger-width out along the lower edges of the sockets. Repeat the pressure. Pause.

8 Continue the pressures at intervals of one finger-width, ending at the points at the outside corners of the sockets.

9 Go back to the inside corners of the sockets and repeat the sequence on the lower ridges one more time.

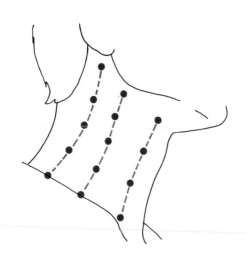

Neck

Kneel at the right side of your partner's upper body, close enough to reach the neck without stretching. The specific points shown in the illustration are only for general guidance. Don't be too concerned with reaching exact points. Just cover the general area as indicated in the illustration. Use the index and middle fingers side by side, and alternate hands, first your right, then your left.

1 Place the index and middle fingers of your right hand side by side under the jaw to the right side of the top of your partner's windpipe. Give light (10-pound) pressure for two seconds, pressing into the muscle, not the windpipe.

2 Place the index and middle fingers of your left hand next to those of your right, on a line made by the windpipe and the neck muscle. Continue down this line to the base of the neck, alternating hands as you go. Give light (10-pound) pressure for two seconds at each point.

3 Bring your hands back up to the top of the neck, slightly further toward the back of the neck, and repeat the pressures, tracing the major neck muscles from the top of the neck to the collarbone, until you have covered the right side of the neck.

4 Move over to your partner's left side and repeat the sequences on the left side of his neck.

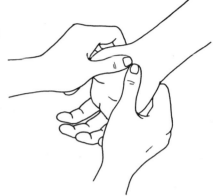

Palms

You give pressure to four points on the palm of each hand. The first three are on the line which runs from the center of the wrist to the base of the middle finger. The fourth is on the heel of the thumb.

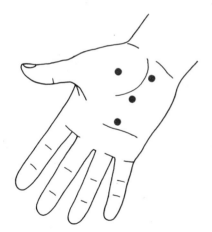

1 Pick up your partner's right hand in both your hands and place your thumbs side by side on the point in the center of the heel of the hand. Give deep (20-pound) pressure for three seconds. Pause.

2 Move down the line to the center of the right palm and repeat the deep pressure for three seconds. Pause.

3 Place your thumbs side by side on the fleshy pad at the base of the middle finger. Repeat the deep (20-pound) pressure.

4 Move your thumbs over to the point on the heel of the thumb and repeat the deep pressure.

5   Go back and repeat the entire sequence once more on the right hand.

6   Repeat the entire sequence twice on the left hand.

Final Exercises

Have your partner rest on his back and stretch his arms, legs and toes while inhaling slowly through the nose. Then have him gradually bring his arms down, relax, and exhale slowly, making a hissing noise through the teeth. This exercise should be repeated five times.

Shiatzu will give immediate relief from nearly every type of headache pain. The most common kinds of headache, those caused by fatigue, tension, overindulgence in food or alcohol, or lack of sleep can be treated effectively with a single shiatzu session. The more severe forms of headache, such as migraine, although they can be temporarily relieved by a single shiatzu treatment, require consistent treatments spaced out over a period of days or even weeks for long-lasting results.

In all headaches, muscles of the head and upper neck become tense and tight. Regardless of the specific trigger cause, the actual pain is a result of a combination of muscle tension and blood vessel constriction. Shiatzu, by relaxing the muscles and priming the flow of blood through the circulatory system, goes directly to the pain areas and gives relief. Points on the head and shoulders are treated first. Then, since restoring good circulation is essential to relaxing muscles, I give pressure to the soles of the feet, the most distant points from the heart. Shiatzu on the soles of the feet improves full-body circulation and directly affects headache pain.

While shiatzu is extremely effective in relieving pain, you should not ignore its great value in preventing the recurrence of pain. If you suffer from frequent headaches, try the shiatzu for headache sequences that follow on a daily basis for a week or so. You will have fewer headaches and when they strike they will be less severe. If you keep up the treatments headaches should eventually disappear entirely. If the headaches don't disappear, you must consult a physician, for they may be caused by organic problems.

Chapter 8

Headaches

SELF-SHIATZU FOR HEADACHES

The exercises which follow can be done while you are sitting in a chair, anytime and anywhere you feel yourself beginning to experience a headache. The full sequence takes only about ten minutes. And if you still suffer discomfort, go back to the areas that gave you the most relief, usually the base of the skull, the back of the neck, the temples and the points around the eyes. If you feel the headache recurring, do the full sequence again. If possible lie down for a few minutes after you finish shiatzu. Close your eyes and breathe deeply.

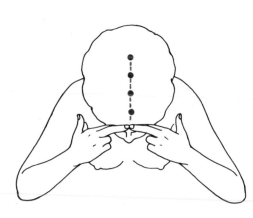

Top of the Head

You should give moderate (15-pound) pressure at points along five lines which run from the front to the back of the head. You should give pressure to points along these lines with the tip of the middle finger of each hand on top of the respective index fingernail.

1 Begin by arching your fingers and placing your index fingers side by side at your widow's peak. Put the tip of the middle finger on top of the nail of each index finger. Give moderate (15-pound) pressure. Hold for three seconds. Pause.

2 Move two finger-widths toward the rear of the crown, along the line of an imaginary center part in your hair. Repeat the moderate pressure. Hold for three seconds. Pause.

3 Continue backward along this imaginary center part at two finger-width intervals, to the midpoint of the rear of the crown. Give moderate (15-pound) pressure at each point for three seconds.

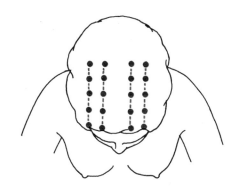

4 Return to the front of your crown and place your left index finger at the point two finger-widths to the left of the widow's peak. Place your right finger two finger-widths to the right. Keep the middle fingers in place on the nails of the index fingers. Give moderate (15-pound) pressure for three seconds. Pause.

5 Give moderate pressure at two finger-width intervals along these lines parallel to a center part in your hair to the rear of the crown. Hold each pressure for three seconds.

6 Return again to the front of your hairline. Move each of your hands two more finger-widths away from the widow's peak. Give moderate (15-pound) pressure at the hairline points. Hold for three seconds. Pause.

7 Repeat the moderate pressure at two finger-width intervals along lines parallel to the previous lines, to the rear of your crown.

Top of the Shoulders

Place the index and middle fingers of your left hand on the top of your right shoulder, halfway between the base of the neck and the edge of the shoulder. Probe slightly to the rear of the shoulder muscle with your fingers. When you are on the most tender spot you have found the point.

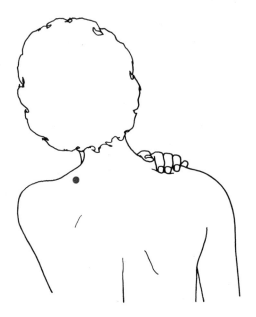

1 Give deep (20-pound) pressure with the index and middle fingers side by side for three seconds. Pause.

2 Repeat the pressure. Pause.

3 Give pressure again for three seconds. Pause.

4 Locate the same point on your left shoulder with the index and middle fingers of your right hand. Repeat the sequence.

Base of the Skull

Using the index and middle fingers of both hands, reach behind your head and place them in the slight indentation at the top center of the neck just below the base of the skull.

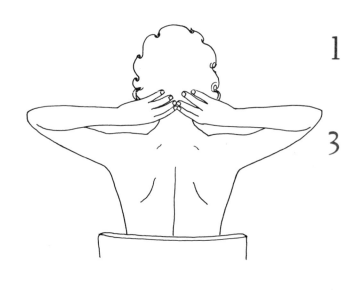

1 Give deep (20-pound) pressure in the recess with the index and middle fingers of both hands.

2 Hold for three seconds. Pause.

3 Repeat the deep pressure two more times. Hold for three seconds each time.

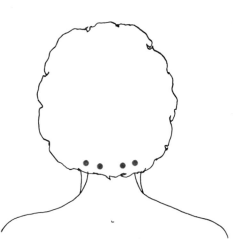

4 Move the index and middle fingers of your left hand three finger-widths to the left along the lower edge of the skull. Move the right index and middle fingers three finger-widths to the right. Give deep (20-pound) pressure at these points simultaneously for three seconds. Repeat two more times.

5 Again move your fingers out three finger-widths along the lower back edge of the skull. Give deep (20-pound) pressure three times. Hold for three seconds each time.

Neck Muscles

Place the index and middle fingers of your left hand at the top of the large muscle which runs down the left outside back of the neck from the base of the skull to the shoulder line. Place your right index and middle fingers on the top of the muscle on the outside right of the back of your neck.

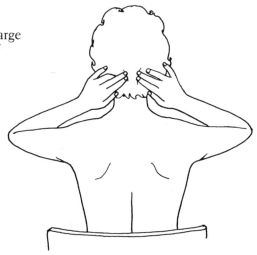

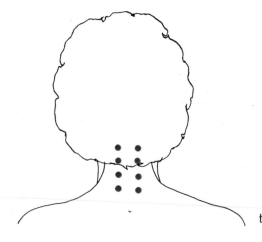

1 Give deep (20-pound) pressure on both points simultaneously for three seconds. Pause.

2 Move down the muscle line approximately two finger-widths. Keep your fingers centered on the muscle bands. Hold for three seconds. Pause.

3 Continue down these muscles giving deep (20-pound) pressure at two finger-width intervals. The final points are at the base of the muscles, on the shoulder line.

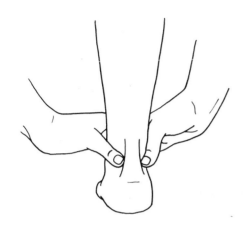

Ankles

Rest your right foot on the floor. Lean forward to work on the ankle. Place your right thumb on the outside of the ankle in the recess between the anklebone and the Achilles tendon which runs into the back of the heel. Place your left thumb on the corresponding point on the inside of the ankle. Then wrap your fingers around the front of the ankle.

1 Give moderate (15-pound) pressure with both thumbs for three seconds. Pause.

2 Move your thumbs down to the inside of the Achilles tendon to the deep recess directly behind the center of the anklebone. Give moderate (15-pound) pressure with both thumbs. Hold for three seconds. Pause.

3 Move down to the recess above the top of the heel. Give moderate pressure with both thumbs. Hold for three seconds.

4 Repeat the sequence on your left ankle, using both thumbs.

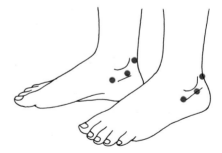

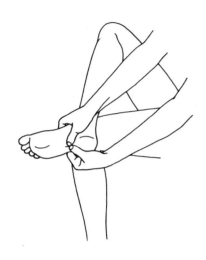

Soles

Place your right leg on your left knee. There are four points on the sole of each foot which should receive pressure. The first three are on a line which bisects the foot from the center of the heel to the center of the middle toe. The fourth point is high in and to the back of the arch slightly above and forward of the first point.

1 Wrap your hands around the top of your foot and place your thumbs side by side just in front of the heel pad. Give deep (20-pound) pressure for three seconds. Pause.

2 Move along the center line to the narrowest part of the foot. Give deep (20-pound) pressure for three seconds. Pause.

3 Move down the center line to the point just behind the ball of the foot. Give deep (20-pound) pressure for three seconds. Pause.

4 Shift your hands and place both thumbs side by side on the point high in the arch. Give deep pressure for three seconds.

5 Place your left leg on your right knee. Repeat the sequence on your left foot.

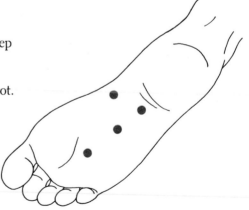

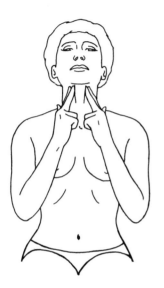

Front and Sides of the Neck

You use the index and middle fingers of both hands on your neck. Although specific points are shown in the illustration you need to use them only for general guidance. Ideally you should cover the neck area, using light to moderate pressure. Do both sides of your neck at the same time.

1 Place the index and middle fingers of your right hand under your jaw at the side of the top of your windpipe. Place the index and middle fingers of your left hand at the corresponding point on the left side. Give light (10-pound) pressure for two seconds. Press down into the muscle, not on the windpipe. Pause.

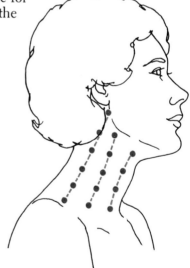

2 Move your fingers down slightly and continue giving light pressure for two seconds at points along the line down to the base of the neck.

3 Bring your hands back to the top of your neck underneath your jaw slightly further along the jawline toward the sides of the neck. Repeat pressures on both sides of your neck along a line descending to the base.

4 Continue the pressures from the top of your neck to the base, each time starting further out to the sides of the neck, until you have covered the front and sides of the neck.

Temples

There are two points on each side of the head. Do corresponding points on both sides simultaneously, with the middle finger of each hand on top of the nail of the index finger.

1   Place your right index and middle fingers on the small recess about two finger-widths beyond the outside corner of your right eye and a little above it. Place the fingers of your left hand on the same point above and out from your left eye.

2   Give moderate (15-pound) pressure for three seconds. Pause.

3   Repeat the moderate pressure. Hold for three seconds. Pause.

4   Move your fingers up and back two finger-widths on a forty-five-degree angle from the initial points. Give moderate (15-pound) pressure. Hold for three seconds. Pause.

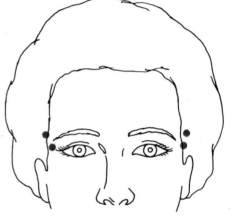

Eyes

The points surrounding your eyes are extremely important in treating a headache. Pressure here relieves built-up pressure on the eye muscles. Use the index, middle and third fingers of your right hand for the points indicated for the right eye, and the corresponding fingers of your left hand for the left eye. Do both eyes at the same time. If you are wearing contact lenses, remove them.

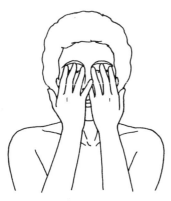

1 Spread your fingers slightly and place the bulbs on the inside of the upper ridge of the eye sockets. The third finger of each hand should be as close to the nose as possible.

2 Give light (10-pound) pressure for three seconds, pressing upward against the inner ridge of the sockets.

3 Draw your fingers down and rest the bulbs on your closed eyelids. Press gently (2 to 3 pounds) for three seconds. Pause.

4 Arch your fingers and press on the inner edge of the lower ridge of the eye sockets. Use light (10-pound) pressure against the bone. Hold for three seconds. Pause.

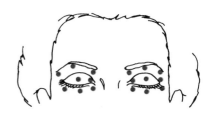

5 Repeat the entire sequence—upper ridge, the eyelids and the lower ridge.

Rest for a few moments when you finish this self-shiatsu. Sit back in your chair and inhale through your nose, filling your lungs with air. Hold the air for three seconds and then exhale slowly through your mouth. Repeat this at least six times.

PARTNER-SHIATZU FOR HEADACHES

The exercises which follow are described with your partner lying flat. If, however, you are giving shiatzu in a place where it is difficult or impossible for your partner to lie flat, for example, in an office, have her sit in a chair while you cover the points that are described. The only difference in giving shiatzu to someone in an upright position is that you must do it with one hand at a time, using your other hand to brace the body so that you can exert sufficient pressure. For instance, when doing the base of the skull or the back of the neck, stand behind your partner, place your left hand on the forehead and give pressure with your right hand. Do the right side of the area first, then the left. At the completion of the shiatzu have your partner close her eyes, breathe deeply, and relax for as long as possible.

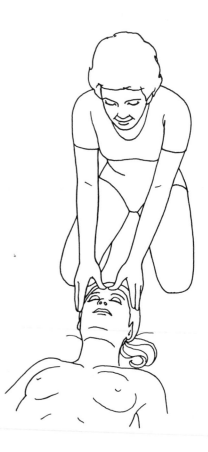

Top of the Head

Begin partner-shiatzu with your partner lying flat on her back on a folded blanket or soft pallet. Kneel beyond the top of your partner's head, close enough so that you can reach the top of the head without stretching.

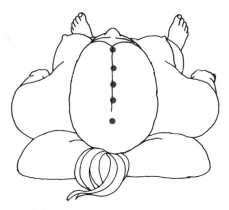

1   Place both thumbs side by side at her widow's peak. Give moderate (15-pound) pressure for three seconds. Pause.

2   Move your thumbs two finger-widths toward the rear of the crown along a line made by a center part in her hair. Give moderate (15-pound) pressure for three seconds. Pause.

3   Continue back to the rear of the crown at two finger-width intervals. Give moderate pressure for three seconds at each point.

4   Move your hands back to the hairline. Place your right thumb two finger-widths out from the widow's peak toward the right side of the head, your left thumb the same distance to the left. Give moderate (15-pound) pressure at these points for three seconds. Pause.

5   Move your thumbs directly back two finger-widths toward the rear of the crown. Give moderate pressure. Hold for three seconds. Pause.

6   Continue giving moderate pressure at two finger-width intervals until you reach the rear of the crown.

7   Come back again to the hairline and move each of your thumbs two finger-widths further out to the sides of the head. Give moderate (15-pound) pressure at two finger-width intervals until you again reach the rear of the crown. Hold for three seconds at each point.

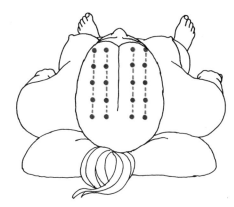

Top of the Shoulders

Have your partner turn over and rest on her stomach. Still kneeling above her head, extend your left arm and place your left thumb on top of her right shoulder. The shoulder point is three or four finger-widths out from the base of the neck. It is next to the knob of bone on top of the shoulder and slightly to the rear.

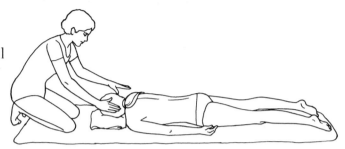

1 Place your right thumbtip on top of your left thumbnail. Give deep (20-pound) pressure to the shoulder point for three seconds. Pause.

2 Repeat the deep pressure two more times. Hold for three seconds each time.

3 Line up above your partner's left shoulder. Reverse the position of your thumbs, placing the left on top of the right. Repeat the pressure sequences on the left shoulder.

Base of the Skull

You must change your position to work effectively on this area. Stand astride her, with your feet on a line just below her hips. Bend down from your waist. (If this is tiring, kneel with your weight resting on your lower legs.)

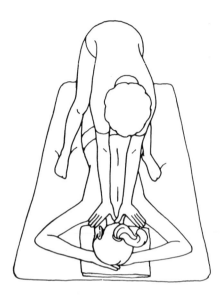

1   Place your right thumb in the recess slightly below the base of the skull, at the top center of the neck. Put your left thumb on top of your right thumbnail. Give deep (20-pound) pressure. Hold for three seconds. Pause.

2   Repeat the pressure two more times. Hold for three seconds each time.

3   Separate your hands and place your left thumb three finger-widths out to the left on the lower back edge of the skull. Move your right thumb three finger-widths out to the right. Give deep (20-pound) pressure with each thumb. Hold for three seconds. Pause.

4   Repeat the pressure two more times. Hold for three seconds each time.

5   Move your thumbs three more finger-widths out along the lower back edge of the skull. Give deep (20-pound) pressure for three seconds. Pause.

6   Repeat the pressure two more times.

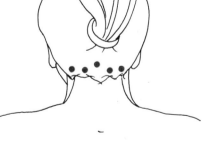

Back of the Neck

Still straddling your partner, place your left thumb at the top of the major muscle which runs down the outside back of the neck. Place your right thumb at the top of the right muscle. Your thumbs should be at the points where the muscles begin at the back of the skull.

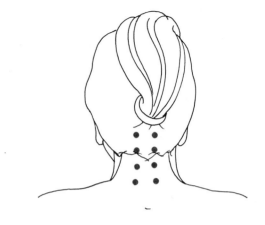

1   Give deep (20-pound) pressure on both points. Hold for three seconds. Pause.

2   Move down the muscle lines two finger-widths. Give deep (20-pound) pressure with your thumbs centered on the muscles. Hold for three seconds. Pause.

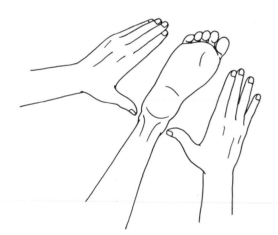

3   Continue down, giving deep (20-pound) pressure at two finger-width intervals. The final points are at the base of the muscle on the shoulder line.

Ankles

You must change your position to work on the ankles. Kneel alongside your partner's right knee, facing the ankle. Place your left thumb on the outside of the ankle, at the top of the recess between the anklebone and the Achilles tendon. Place your right thumb on the corresponding point at the inside of the ankle. Wrap your fingers around the front of the ankle.

1   Give moderate (15-pound) pressure with both thumbs. Hold for three seconds. Pause.

2   Repeat the pressure for three seconds.

3   Move both thumbs down inside the Achilles tendon to the deep recess between the back of the anklebone and the tendon. Give moderate (15-pound) pressure. Hold for three seconds. Pause. Then repeat the pressure for three seconds.

4   Move your thumbs down to the recess above the top of the heel. Give moderate pressure for three seconds. Pause. Repeat the pressure.

5   Move to your partner's left side and repeat the sequences on her left ankle.

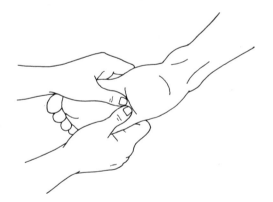

Soles

Move back to a position below your partner's right foot. Four points on the sole of each foot should receive pressure. The first three are on a line which bisects the foot. The fourth is high in and to the back of the arch, above and slightly forward of the first point.

1   Wrap your fingers around the top of the right foot. Place your thumbs side by side just in front of the center of the heel pad. Give deep (20-pound) pressure for three seconds. Pause.

2 Move down the line to the center of the foot. Give deep (20-pound) pressure for three seconds. Pause.

3 Move down the line to the point just behind the center of the ball of the foot. Give deep pressure for three seconds. Pause.

4 Shift your hands and place both thumbs side by side on the point high in the arch. Give deep pressure for three seconds.

5 Move to your partner's left foot and repeat the sequence.

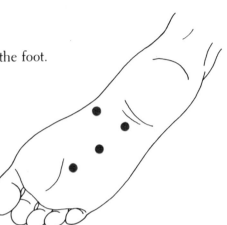

When you have finished with the sole of the left foot, have your partner turn over and rest on her back. This will be her position for the final shiatzu for headache exercises.

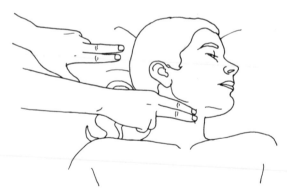

Neck

Kneel to the right of your partner's upper body. You should be able to reach her neck comfortably without stretching your arms. Although specific points are shown in the illustration, you need to use them only as a general guide. The idea is to cover the neck area thoroughly. Just cover the general area, starting beneath the jaw and working down to the base of the neck. Use the index and middle fingers of both hands, alternating your right and left hands.

1 Place the index and middle fingers of your right hand under the jaw beside the top of the windpipe. Give light (10-pound) pressure at the top of a line made by the side of the windpipe and the muscle. Be careful not to press directly on the windpipe, but into the muscle. Hold for two seconds. Pause.

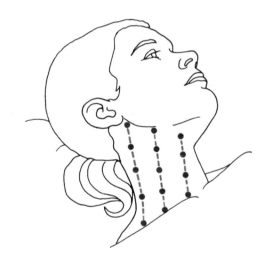

2 Place the index and middle fingers of your left hand just below the point you have just pressed with your right hand. Repeat the light pressure.

3 Continue to move straight down alongside the windpipe, alternating your hands to give light pressure, until you reach the base of the neck.

4 Bring your hands back up to the top of the neck under the jaw. Repeat the pressures, alternating your hands, along a descending line to the base of the neck.

5 Continue the light (10-pound) pressures from the top of the neck to the base until you have covered the right side of the neck.

6 Move to your partner's left side and repeat the sequences on the left side of the neck.

Temples

Move back to your position above your partner's head. There are two points on each side of the head. Use the index and middle fingers of each hand to do both sides of the head simultaneously.

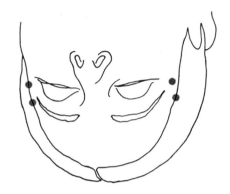

1 Give moderate (15-pound) pressure in the recesses of the temple. Hold for three seconds. Pause.

2 Repeat the moderate pressure. Hold for three seconds. Pause.

3 Move your fingers up to the hairline to the muscle that moves when you clench your teeth. Give moderate (15-pound) pressure for three seconds. Pause.

4 Repeat the moderate pressure. Hold for three seconds.

Eyes

The points around the eyes are on the inside edges of the eye sockets. Use the index fingers of both hands and do the points on the right and left eyes simultaneously.

1 Place your index fingers on the inner edge of the upper ridges of the sockets, as close to the nose as possible.

2 Give light (10-pound) pressure directly on the inner edge of the socket bones for three seconds. Pause.

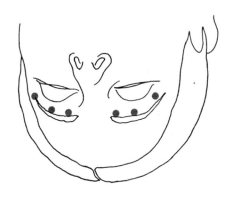

3 Move your fingers one finger-width toward the outsides of the eyes, keeping your fingers on the inner edge of the socket bones. Repeat the light pressure for three seconds. Pause.

4 Continue the pressures at consistent one finger-width intervals along the socket bones until you have covered the points around the tops of the eyes.

5 Reposition yourself, if necessary, in order to reach the points on the lower ridges of the eye sockets. Kneel close to your partner's midsection.

6 Give light (10-pound) pressure directly on the inner edge of the bone adjacent to the nose. Hold for three seconds. Pause.

7 Move your fingers out along the lower edge of the sockets one finger-width. Repeat the light pressure for three seconds. Pause.

8 Continue the pressure at one finger-width intervals until you have covered the points along the lower ridges of the sockets.

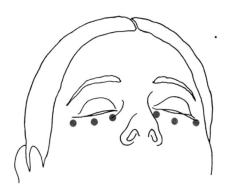

Partner–Shiatzu 177

Final Exercises

Have your partner extend her arms out on the floor above her head. Grip her hands and pull gently, stretching her arms. At the same time your partner should inhale through her nose, filling her lungs to capacity, while stretching her legs and toes. Hold a moment, then release the tension on her hands while she exhales slowly through her mouth, relaxing her whole body. Repeat this exercise six times.

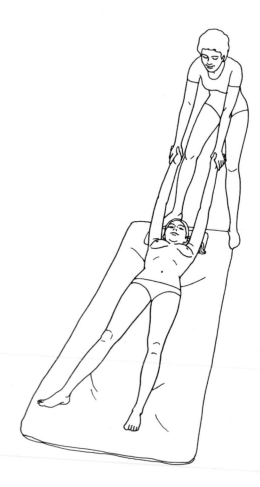

Through shiatzu you can easily rid yourself of stiffness and pain of the neck and shoulders caused by fatigue, nervous tension and physical overexertion.

Many people who are high-strung or who have a lot of nervous energy have come to me with severe tightness through the neck and shoulder muscles. Often this pain is the result of the unconscious accumulation of tension over months or even years. Yet without exception these people have gained relief and a sense of relaxation after my first treatment of shiatzu.

The specific exercises which I give for neck and shoulder stiffness caused by tension are equally effective for people who have strained their muscles through physical overexertion. Of course, when you or your partner suffer shoulder or neck soreness and stiffness shiatzu should be given as soon as possible. If any pain or soreness begins to return, the sequences should be repeated. Even if there is no residue of stiffness on the following day, I feel that the shiatzu exercises should once again be repeated.

The first pressures are given to the head and neck. These pressures begin to open the pathways between the head and the heart. The tops of the shoulders and the upper back and shoulder blades are next. These areas, although probably painful at first to your touch, must receive steady and deep pressures. Shiatzu's priming action releases the tension and hastens a steady flow of blood to the troubled areas. Then I give light pressure on the sides and front of the neck, and finally, deep pressure up into the armpits, along the upper arms and on the lower front of the shoulders.

Chapter 9

Stiff Neck
and
Sore
Shoulders

SELF-SHIATZU FOR STIFF NECK AND SORE SHOULDERS

This self-shiatzu sequence is designed to be done while you are sitting in a straight-backed chair.

Top and Back of the Head

Place the index and middle fingers of both hands together at the top of your crown.

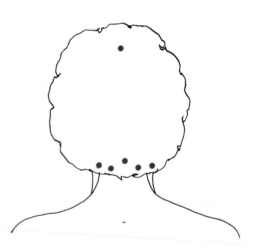

1 Give deep (20-pound) pressure for three seconds. Pause. Repeat the pressure.

2 Move your hands down to the recess at the center of the base of the skull, where the top of the neck joins the skull. Give deep pressure with the index and middle fingers of both hands. Hold the pressure for three seconds. Pause.

3 Separate your hands and place the index and middle fingers of each hand two finger-widths to either side of the center of the rear of the head, just below the bottom ridge of the skull. Give deep (20-pound) pressure for three seconds. Pause.

4 Move each of your hands two finger-widths further out along the bottom ridge of the skull. Repeat the deep pressure.

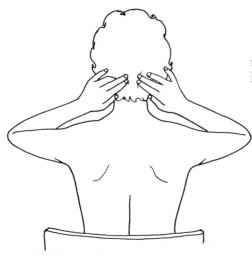

Back of the Neck

Place the index and middle fingers of each hand at the top of the large muscles which run down the back of the neck from the base of the skull. Place the fingers of the left hand at the top of the left muscle, at the top of the muscle band, and the fingers of the right hand at the corresponding point on the right side.

1 Give deep (20-pound) pressure on both points simultaneously for three seconds. Pause.

2 Move halfway down the muscle line and repeat the deep pressure. Pause.

3 Move down to the base of the muscle line, where the neck meets the shoulder. Repeat the deep pressure once more.

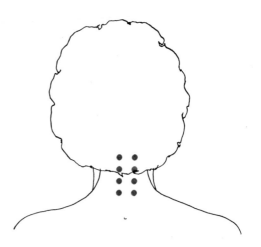

Shoulders

Find the point on top of your right shoulder with the index and middle fingers of your left hand. The point is halfway between the base of the neck and the edge of your shoulder. Probe slightly to the rear of the shoulder muscle with your fingers. When you are on the most tender spot you have found the point.

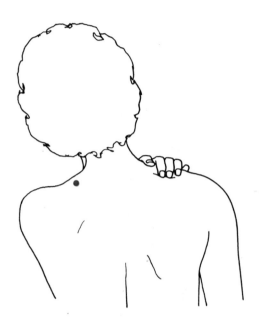

1   Give deep (20-pound) pressure for three seconds. Pause.

2   Find the corresponding point on your left shoulder with the fingers of your right hand. Repeat the deep pressure for three seconds.

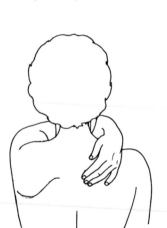

Upper Back and Shoulder Blades

Extend your left hand over your right shoulder and down your back as far as you can reach. Place the index, middle and third fingers of your right hand next to the spine so that the index finger is just beside the vertebrae.

1   Give deep (20-pound) pressure for three seconds. Pause.

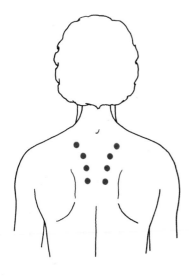

2   Move your hands two finger-widths straight up the line toward the shoulder. Repeat the deep pressure for three seconds. Pause.

3   Continue up the line at two finger-width intervals until you reach the shoulder line, giving deep (20-pound) pressure at each point.

4   Reach your left hand over your right shoulder and place the index, middle and third fingers of the left hand on the upper edge of the shoulder blade at the inside corner. Give deep pressure for three seconds.

5   Extend your right hand over your left shoulder and reach down as far as you can on your back. Repeat the first sequence (steps 1 to 3) on the left side of your upper back.

6   Reach your right hand over your left shoulder and repeat the second sequence (step 4) at the corresponding point on your left shoulder blade.

Front and Sides of the Neck

Use the index and middle fingers of both hands to give shiatzu to the points on the neck, the left hand for the left side of the neck and the right hand for the right side. Although specific points are shown in the illustration, they are only for general guidance. You should cover the entire neck area with light to moderate pressure. Press corresponding points on both sides simultaneously.

1 Place the index and middle fingers of your right hand under your jaw at the top of the line made by the neck muscle and the windpipe. Do the same on the left side with your left hand. Give light (10-pound) pressure for two seconds. Pause.

2 Move your fingers down slightly and repeat the pressure. Pause.

3 Continue down the line to the base of the neck, giving light pressure for two seconds at each point.

4 Bring your hands back up to the top of the neck and repeat the pressures, tracing the major neck muscles from the top to the base of the neck until you have covered the sides of the neck.

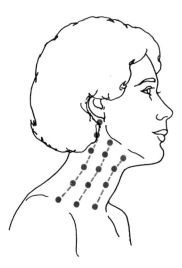

Arms and Shoulders

The first point in this final sequence is deep in the armpit. Then there are three points on the outside of the arm starting at the top nearest the shoulder, then finally, three points running diagonally down the front of the shoulder.

1   Lift your right arm and place your left thumb deep into your right armpit. Give deep (20-pound) pressure for two seconds. Pause.

2   Place the index and middle fingers of your left hand at the top of the outside corner of your right shoulder. Give deep (20-pound) pressure for two seconds. Pause.

3   Move your fingers two finger-widths down the outside of the upper arm. Repeat the deep pressure for two seconds. Pause.

4   Move two finger-widths further down and repeat the pressure.

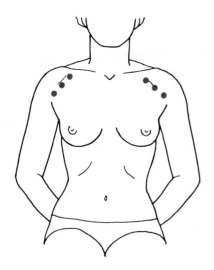

5   Place the index and middle fingers of your left hand in the hollow under the outer end of your collarbone. Give deep (20-pound) pressure for two seconds. Pause.

6   Move your fingers two finger-widths diagonally in the direction of your armpit and repeat the deep pressure. Pause.

7   Move your fingers two finger-widths further in the direction of your armpit and repeat the deep pressure.

8   Change hands and repeat the sequence (steps 1 to 7) on the corresponding points on your left side.

Final Exercises

Rest for a few moments when you finish this self-shiatzu. Sit back in your chair and inhale through your nose, filling your lungs with air. Hold the air for three seconds and then exhale slowly through your mouth. Repeat this exercise at least six times.

PARTNER-SHIATZU FOR STIFF NECK AND SORE SHOULDERS

Top of the Head and Central Shoulder Points

Begin this sequence with your partner lying on her stomach. You should be kneeling above your partner's head, close enough to reach the tops of her shoulders.

The first point is at the crown of the head. The next two points are at the tops of the shoulders.

1 Place your right thumb on the point at the top of the crown and place your left thumb on top of the right. Give deep (20-pound) pressure for three seconds in the direction of the spine. Pause.

2 Extend your left arm and place your thumb at the center of the top of the right shoulder. The shoulder point is three or four finger-widths out from the base of the neck. It is next to the knob of bone on top of the shoulder and slightly to the rear. Place your right thumb on top of your left thumbnail and give deep (20-pound) pressure for three seconds. Pause. Repeat the pressure.

3 Shift your body so you are lined up above your partner's left shoulder. Place your right thumb on the corresponding shoulder point, and the left thumb on top of the right thumbnail. Give deep (20-pound) pressure for three seconds. Pause. Repeat the pressure.

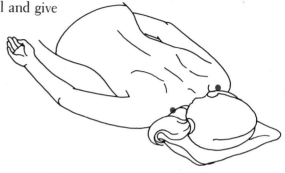

Base of the Skull

Stand or kneel astride your partner, so that you can reach her neck easily, and place your thumbs side by side at the top center of the neck in the recess just below the base of the skull.

1 Give deep (20-pound) pressure for three seconds. Pause.

2 Move both thumbs out two finger-widths to the right, just below the bottom ridge of the skull, and repeat the deep (20-pound) pressure. Pause.

3 Move your thumbs two finger-widths further out to the right just below the bottom ridge of the skull. Give deep pressure.

4 Move over to the left, two finger-widths to the side of the center of the base of the skull. Give deep (20-pound) pressure with both thumbs. Hold for three seconds. Pause.

5 Move two finger-widths further to the left just below the bottom edge of the skull. Repeat the deep pressure.

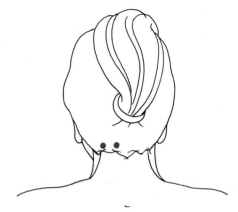

Back of the Neck

Separate your hands and place your thumbs at the top of the major muscles which run down the back of the neck. Place your left thumb at the top of the left muscle, just below the bottom of the skull, and the right thumb at the corresponding point on the right side.

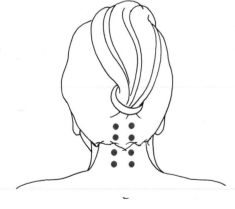

1 Give deep (20-pound) pressure on both points for three seconds. Pause.

2 Move down the muscle lines two finger-widths. Repeat the deep pressure. Pause.

3 Continue down the muscle lines, giving deep (20-pound) pressure at two finger-width intervals, ending at the base of the muscles on the shoulder line.

Upper Back

Still straddling your partner, place your left thumb immediately to the right of the spine, just below the big bulging vertebra at the base of the neck. Place your right thumb two finger-widths further to the right on the same line.

1   Give moderate (15-pound) pressure with both thumbs for three seconds. Pause.

2   Move two finger-widths straight down along the side of the spine and repeat the moderate pressure with both thumbs. Pause.

3   Continue down the right side of the spine at two finger-width intervals until you are on a line with the center of the shoulder blade.

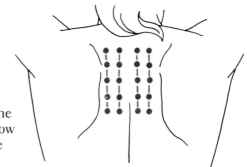

4   Move back up to the top of the spine, placing your right thumb immediately to the left of the spine, just below the major vertebra at the base of the neck, and the left thumb two finger-widths further to the left. Follow the previous sequence (steps 1 to 3) to a point on a line with the middle of the shoulder blade.

Shoulder Blades and Joints

The point on the shoulder blades is just under the ridge that runs along the top of the shoulder blades, on the corner that is closest to the spine. The point on the joints is in the corner of the angle formed by the shoulder and the upper arm bone. Press both points on the right side before those on the left.

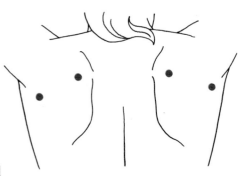

1 Place your left thumb under the ridge of the right shoulder blade, at the inside edge of the corner close to the spine. At the same time grasp the right shoulder with your right hand. Give deep (20-pound) pressure for three seconds with your left thumb. Pause.

2 Move your left thumb over to the corner of the angle formed by the shoulder and the upper arm bone. Keep your hold with your right hand on the shoulder. Give deep (20-pound) pressure with your left thumb.

3 Reverse hands and repeat the pressures on the corresponding points on the left side.

Neck

This sequence and all that follow cover the neck and the shoulder areas. Perform all the sequences on the right side, then move over to your partner's left side and repeat the sequences on the left side.

Have your partner turn over and rest on her back. Kneel to the right of her upper body. You should be able to reach her neck comfortably without stretching your arms. Although specific points are shown in the illustration, you need to use them only as a general guide. The idea is to cover the neck area thoroughly. Just cover the general area, starting beneath the jaw and working down to the base of the neck. Use the index and middle fingers of both hands, alternating your right and left hands.

1 Place the index and middle fingers of your right hand under the jaw beside the top of the windpipe. Give light (10-pound) pressure at the top of a line made by the side of the windpipe and the muscle. Be careful not to press directly on the windpipe, but into the muscle. Hold for two seconds. Pause.

2 Place the index and middle fingers of your left hand just below the point you have just pressed with your right hand. Repeat the light pressure.

3 Continue to move straight down alongside the windpipe, alternating your hands, giving light pressure until you reach the base of the neck.

4 Bring your hands back up to the top of the neck under the jaw. Repeat the pressures, alternating your hands, along a descending line to the base of the neck.

5 Continue the light (10-pound) pressures from the top of the neck to the base until you have covered the right side of the neck.

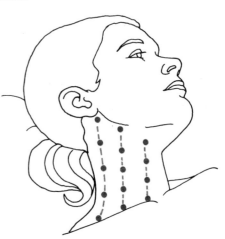

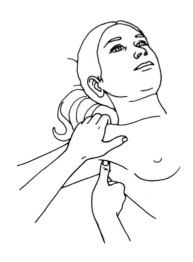

Armpit and Shoulder

The first point in this sequence is deep in the armpit.
Then three points run diagonally down the front of the shoulder.
Finally, three points run down the outside of the arm, starting
at the top corner of the shoulder.

1 Grasp the corner of your partner's right
shoulder with your left hand and
place your right thumb deep in the armpit.
Give deep (20-pound) pressure for two seconds.
Pause. Repeat the pressure.

2 Cross the tip of your right middle finger
over the nail of the index finger.
Keep your grasp on your partner's shoulder and
place your fingers in the hollow under the outer
end of your partner's collarbone. Give deep
(20-pound) pressure for two seconds. Pause.

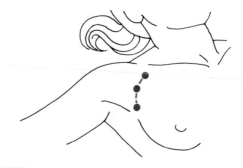

3 Move your fingers two finger-widths diagonally out and down in the direction of your partner's armpit and repeat the deep pressure. Pause.

4 Move your fingers two finger-widths further in the direction of the armpit and repeat the deep pressure.

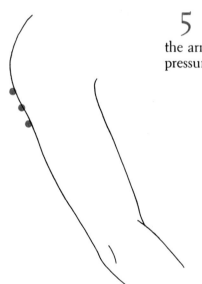

5 Place your thumbs side by side at the top of the outside of your partner's shoulder. Wrap your hands around the upper arm, with your fingers curved around to the armpit. Give deep (20-pound) pressure for two seconds. Pause. Repeat the pressure.

6 Move your thumbs two finger-widths down the outside of the upper arm. Repeat the deep pressure. Pause. Repeat the pressure.

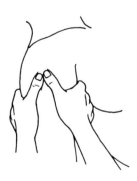

7 Move two finger-widths further down and repeat the pressure. Pause. Repeat the pressure.

Move over and kneel at the left side of your partner's upper body. Repeat the neck sequence and the armpit-and-shoulder sequence on the corresponding points on the left side.

Final Exercises

Have your partner extend her arms out on the floor above her head. Grip her hands and pull gently, stretching her arms. At the same time she should inhale through her nose, filling her lungs to capacity, while stretching her legs and toes. Hold a moment, then release the tension on her hands while she exhales slowly through her mouth, relaxing her whole body. Repeat this exercise six times.

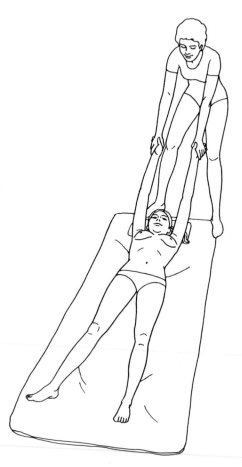

Shiatzu can give you quick and effective relief from lower back pains caused by tension or muscle strain. While as a professional I have treated backaches caused by all sorts of spinal problems, I must stress to you that *severe or chronic conditions such as slipped disks or organic degeneration should be treated only by professionals working closely with physicians.*

The lower back problems which you or your friends are most likely to encounter come as a result of physical strain or emotional stress. The special shiatzu sequences which I have developed will, if applied as soon as possible after the pain begins, free you from serious discomfort.

Over the years I have worked closely with many dancers and athletes. To many of them frequent straining of the lower back is an accepted although unwelcome occupational hazard. Shiatzu has constantly made it possible for them to resume performing at the height of their capacity.

I always recommend that this shiatzu sequence be repeated at least twice at daily intervals. Of course treatment should be repeated immediately if and when pain returns. But even if there is no tightening or soreness after the first shiatzu, repeat the full sequence within twenty-four hours.

For low back pain I concentrate on the spine and the areas adjacent to the spine, then the abdomen. In combination, pressure on these areas serves to relax the muscular complex of the lower body. If the pain is severe, repeat the entire sequence and also give shiatzu to the upper back and shoulders as well. (See Chapter 5, pp. 72–74, for these self-shiatzu exercises; Chapter 6, pp. 96–100, for partner-shiatzu.)

Chapter 10

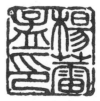

Low Back Pain

SELF-SHIATZU FOR LOW BACK PAIN

These exercises are designed to be done while you are sitting in a chair.

Lower Back

Sit forward in your chair so that you can reach the sides of the lower spine. The points on the lower back run from the fleshy area midway down the buttocks up alongside the spine as far as you can reach. The sequence ends with a pair of points out on the waistline. Press corresponding points on both sides simultaneously.

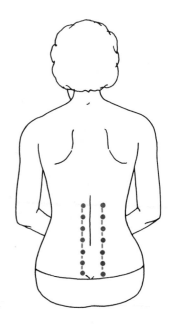

1   Place the index, middle and third fingers of both hands on the buttocks at the bottom of the spine, with the third finger of each hand one finger-width to either side of the spine. Give deep (20-pound) pressure for three seconds. Pause.

2   Move both hands two finger-widths up the spine and repeat the deep pressure. Pause.

3   Continue up alongside the spine at two finger-width intervals. Give deep pressure for three seconds at each point. Keep the third finger of each hand a finger-width to the side of the spine.

4   Repeat this sequence (steps 1 to 3) two more times.

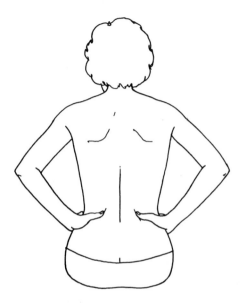

5 Rest your fingers on the tops of your hipbones and extend your thumbs in toward the spine at the waistline. Locate each thumb three finger-widths out from the center of the spine, directly on the waistline.

6 Give deep (20-pound) pressure with both thumbs simultaneously for three seconds. Pause.

7 Repeat this pressure at least two more times. This is usually the most tense point, so press here until you feel it relax.

Abdomen

At this point you may lie down, if you can. It is more relaxing and you can press deeper. Otherwise, remain seated, but lean back into the chair.

The points on the abdomen run down three lines along the abdomen. The first line runs down the center of the abdomen; the last two lines (a pair) run parallel to it on either side of the trunk.

1 Place the index, middle and third fingers of both hands side by side just below the center of the rib cage. Give moderate (15-pound) pressure for three seconds. Pause.

2 Move both hands two finger-widths down the center line and repeat the moderate pressure. Pause.

3 Continue down the center line at two finger-width intervals, giving moderate pressure for three seconds at each point, until you reach the top of the pubic bone.

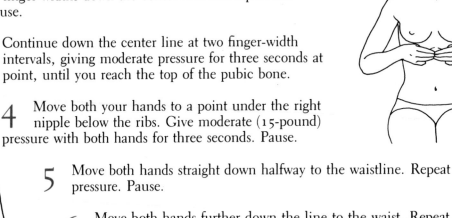

4 Move both your hands to a point under the right nipple below the ribs. Give moderate (15-pound) pressure with both hands for three seconds. Pause.

5 Move both hands straight down halfway to the waistline. Repeat the moderate pressure. Pause.

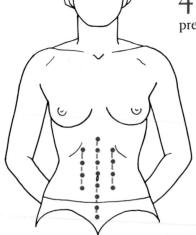

6 Move both hands further down the line to the waist. Repeat the moderate pressure. Pause.

7 Move to the point midway between the waistline and the groin. Give moderate (15-pound) pressure for three seconds two more times.

8 Move your hands over to the corresponding point on the left side of the abdomen and repeat the sequence (steps 4 to 7) on the corresponding points on the left side.

9 Place your palms on your abdomen. Give light (10-pound) and even pressure with both palms simultaneously. Move your palms so that you cover your abdomen with gentle pressure. Concentrate on areas where the muscles feel most tense until they relax.

Final Exercises

Rest for a few moments when you finish this self-shiatzu. Sit back in your chair and inhale through your nose, filling your lungs with air. Hold the air for three seconds and then exhale slowly through your mouth. Repeat this exercise at least six times.

PARTNER-SHIATZU FOR LOW BACK PAIN

Bottom of the Spine

Your partner should lie on her stomach on the floor cushioned by a folded blanket, her head resting on her hands on a folded towel. Straddle her so that you can easily reach the lower half of her spine. If you run your thumb down the spine you can feel the recesses between the vertebrae. You apply the pressure in these recesses, alternating thumbs, all the way from above the waistline to the bottom of the spine. Give pressure with your arms extended and the weight of your upper body transmitted down to and through your thumbs.

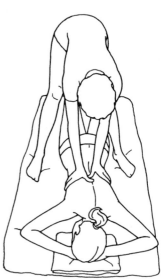

Partner–Shiatzu 199

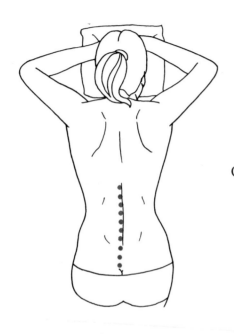

1 Place your right thumb in the recess four or five finger-widths above the waistline. Give moderate (15-pound) pressure for three seconds. Pause.

2 Place your left thumb in the next lower recess down the spine. Repeat the moderate pressure. Pause.

3 Continue down the spine to the tailbone, alternating thumbs. Give moderate pressure at each point.

4 Repeat the above sequence (steps 1 to 3) two more times.

Right and Left Sides of the Spine

Without changing your position, place your left thumb immediately to the right of the spine, five finger-widths above the waistline. Place your right thumb two finger-widths further to the right.

1 Give moderate (15-pound) pressure with both thumbs for three seconds. Pause.

2 Move both thumbs two finger-widths straight down alongside the spine. Repeat the pressure. Pause.

3 Continue down the side of the spine at two finger-width intervals. Give moderate (15-pound) pressure for three seconds at each point, pause, then continue, ending at a point midway down the buttock.

4 Repeat the above sequence (steps 1 to 3) two more times.

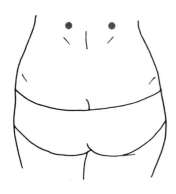

5 Move over to your partner's right side. Place your left thumbtip on top of your right thumbtip on a point on the waistline on top of the big muscle band that runs parallel to the spine. Give deep (20-pound) pressure, pressing toward the spine. Pause.

6 Repeat the pressure at least two more times. This is usually the most tense point, so repeat the pressure until you feel the tension relax.

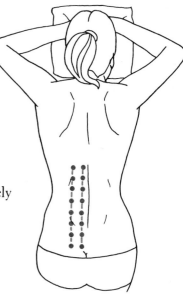

7 Move back to a position astride your partner, placing your right thumb immediately to the left of the spine, four or five finger-widths above the waistline. Place your left thumb two finger-widths further to the left. Repeat the first sequence (steps 1 to 4) on the points running down alongside the spine.

8 Move over to your partner's left side and repeat the second sequence (steps 5 to 6) on the left hip/waist point.

Abdomen

Have your partner turn over and rest on her back. Kneel next to your partner's right hip so that you can reach the abdomen from the bottom of the rib cage down to the tops of the legs. The points on the abdomen run down three lines from the bottom of the rib cage to the tops of the legs.

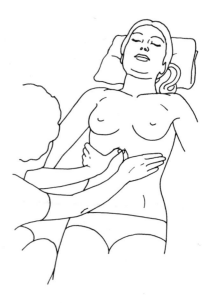

1 Place both thumbs side by side just below the center of the rib cage. Give moderate (15-pound) pressure for three seconds. Pause.

2 Move two finger-widths down the center line and repeat the moderate pressure. Pause.

3 Continue down the center line at two finger-width intervals, giving moderate pressure for three seconds at each point, until you reach the top of the pubic bone.

4 Separate your thumbs and place one below each nipple just below the ribs. Give moderate (15-pound) pressure simultaneously on both the left and right sides for three seconds. Pause.

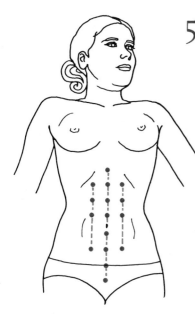

5 Move both thumbs straight down halfway to the waistline. Repeat the moderate pressure. Pause.

6 Move both thumbs further down the lines to the waistline. Repeat the moderate pressure. Pause.

7 Move to the points midway between the waist and the groin. Give moderate pressure for three seconds.

Kneel at your partner's side. Place both hands on her abdomen, palms down. Give light and even (10-pound) pressure with both palms simultaneously, moving your hands to cover the abdomen with gentle pressure. Concentrate on the areas where the muscles feel most tense until you feel some relaxation.

Final Exercises

Have your partner extend her arms out on the floor above her head. Grip her hands and pull gently, stretching her arms. At the same time she should inhale through her nose, filling her lungs to capacity, while stretching her legs and toes. Hold a moment, then release the tension on her hands while she exhales slowly through her mouth, relaxing her whole body. Repeat this exercise six times.

Chapter 11

Constipation and Diarrhea

Shiatzu can relieve you of the discomforts of constipation and diarrhea caused by nervous tension and emotional stress. It will relax your digestive and intestinal tracts and return your system to the balance that assures healthy bowels.

The shiatzu exercises I recommend are the same for both diarrhea and constipation. This is because the problems, although opposite in fact, indicate malfunction of the same system.

Although both problems react to the same treatment, their symptoms are quite different. Constipation usually develops gradually and often becomes chronic in people who are extremely tense. When people suffer from constipation I can always feel a large hard lump to the left of the navel. This is a lump of feces which has become attached to the intestinal wall. Because of nervous tension the regular contraction and dilation of the colon has become retarded, causing the feces to become immobilized. With shiatzu the regular muscle movement of the colon is restored and body waste is eliminated.

A daily shiatzu treatment will be necessary to return your system to normal. How long it will take to correct the problem depends completely on the individual and how long-standing the problem is, but you should have results within a week to ten days.

The onset of diarrhea is more sudden, and its appearance more intermittent, in people experiencing emotional anxiety. It is caused when the muscular movement of the colon, instead of remaining regular and consistent, becomes spasmodic. Shiatzu pressure, which restores the circulatory and muscle systems to normal functioning, effectively remedies this. You will probably find that it requires two or three applications of shiatzu on a daily basis. If the problem recurs after several days, repeat the exercises. You will find that the recurrence becomes less and less frequent.

Warning: Never apply abdominal shiatzu to anyone who is suffering from ulcers or any other abdominal disease or ailment. Do not give this treatment to anyone experiencing tenderness or pain anywhere in the abdomen, or to anyone having even a slight degree of fever. Furthermore, shiatzu will be ineffective, though not harmful, in anyone suffering from diarrhea caused by such external agents as tainted food or a virus.

In the following shiatzu exercises for constipation and diarrhea, pressure is first given to major points of the head and neck. This minimizes the nervous tension and relaxes the brain. The lower back is next, to further relieve tenseness. Then comes shiatzu on the abdomen, the most important area for treatment. Pressure should be given throughout the abdominal area until the tight muscles become completely relaxed.

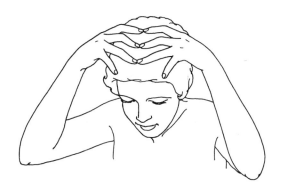

SELF-SHIATZU FOR CONSTIPATION OR DIARRHEA

Head

You can do this entire shiatzu sequence while sitting in a chair. Place the index and middle fingers of both hands together at the top of your crown.

1 Give deep (20-pound) pressure for three seconds. Pause.

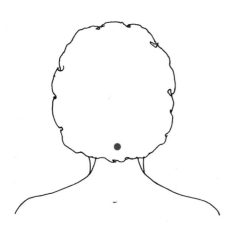

2 Repeat the deep pressure. Pause.

3 Repeat the deep pressure again. Pause.

4 Move your hands down to the hollow at the base of the skull, where the top of the neck joins the skull. Give deep (20-pound) pressure with the index and middle fingers of both hands. Hold the pressure for three seconds. Pause.

5 Repeat the pressure two more times.

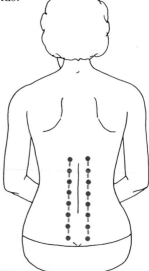

Lower Back

Sit forward in your chair so that you can reach the bottom of the spine. The points on the lower back run from the fleshy area at the top of the buttocks up alongside the spine to the mid-back, as far as you can reach. Press corresponding points on both sides simultaneously.

1 Place the index, middle and third fingers of both hands at the bottom of the spine, with the third finger of the right hand one finger-width to the right of the spine and the third finger of the left hand one finger-width to the left of the spine. Give deep (20-pound) pressure for three seconds. Pause.

2 Move both hands two finger-widths up and repeat the pressure. Pause.

3 Continue up the sides of the spine at two finger-width intervals, keeping the third finger of each hand a finger-width to the side of the spine.

4 Repeat the sequence two more times.

Hips

Sit forward in your chair. Rest your fingers on the tops of your hipbones and extend your thumbs in toward the spine at the waistline. Place each thumb three finger-widths out from the center of the spine, directly on the waistline.

1 Give deep (20-pound) pressure with both thumbs simultaneously for three seconds. Pause.

2 Repeat the deep pressure. Pause.

3 Repeat the pressure again. Pause.

4 Put your hands on your hipbones and move your thumbs down as far as you can toward your buttocks. Locate the points just above the fleshiest part of the buttocks. Give deep (20-pound) pressure on each point with both thumbs simultaneously. Pause.

5 Repeat the deep pressure two more times.

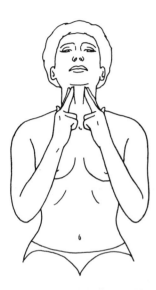

Front and Sides of Neck

For the points on the neck, use the index and middle fingers of both hands, the left hand for the left side of the neck and the right hand for the right side. Although specific points are shown in the illustration, they are just for general guidance. The idea is to cover the neck area with light to moderate pressure. Press corresponding points on both sides simultaneously.

1   Place the index and middle fingers of your right hand under your jaw at the top of the line made by the neck muscle and your windpipe. Do the same on the left side with your left hand. Give light (10-pound) pressure for two seconds. Press down into the muscle, not the windpipe. Pause.

2   Move your fingers down slightly and repeat the pressure. Pause.

3   Continue down the line to the base of the neck, giving light pressure at each point for two seconds.

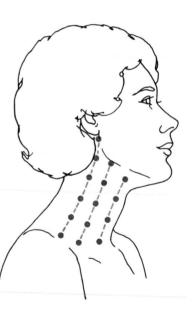

4   Bring your hands back up to the top of the neck slightly further along the jawline toward each side of the neck. Repeat the pressures on both sides of your neck along a line descending to the base.

5   Continue the pressures from the top of the neck to the base, each time starting further out to the sides of the neck, until you have covered the front and sides of the neck.

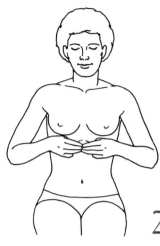

Abdomen

Lean back in your chair. The points on the abdomen run vertically down five lines along the abdomen, between the bottom of the rib cage and the groin. The first line runs down the center of the abdomen. Then a pair of lines runs down either side of the center line. Finally, there is a pair of lines still further out from the center line. After going down the center line, press the points on the right side before proceeding to those on the left.

1 Place the index, middle and third fingers of both hands side by side just below the breastbone in the center of the rib cage. Give moderate (15-pound) pressure for three seconds. Pause.

2 Move down the center line two finger-widths and repeat the moderate pressure. Pause.

3 Continue down the center line at two finger-width intervals, giving moderate pressure for three seconds at each point, until you reach the groin.

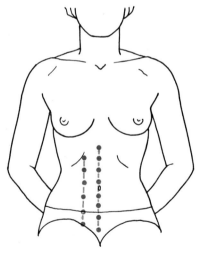

4 Move your hands over four finger-widths to the right of the center line. Place the index, middle and third fingers of both hands just below the bottom rib. Give moderate (15-pound) pressure for three seconds. Pause.

5 Proceed down the line at two finger-width intervals, as above, giving moderate pressure at each point for three seconds, until you reach the base of the trunk.

6 Move your hands over four finger-widths further to the right. Place the index, middle and third fingers of both hands directly below the bottom rib. Give moderate (15-pound) pressure for three seconds. Pause.

7 Continue down the line at two finger-width intervals, giving moderate pressure for three seconds at each point, until you reach the fold at the top of the leg.

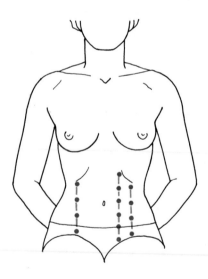

8 Now move over to the left side, four finger-widths from the center line, and place the index, middle and third fingers of both hands just below the bottom rib. Give moderate (15-pound) pressure for three seconds. Pause.

9 Continue down the line at two finger-width intervals, giving moderate pressure for three seconds at each point, until you reach the base of the trunk.

10 Now move four finger-widths further to the left and repeat the same series of pressures at two finger-width intervals, until you reach the fold at the top of the leg.

11 Finally, place both your palms on your abdomen. Give light (10-pound) pressure with both palms simultaneously. Move your palms so that you cover your abdomen with gentle pressure. Concentrate on any areas that feel tense until they relax.

Final Exercises

Rest for a few moments when you finish this self-shiatzu. Sit back in your chair and inhale through your nose, filling your lungs with air. Hold the air for three seconds and then exhale slowly through your mouth. Repeat this exercise at least six times.

PARTNER-SHIATZU FOR CONSTIPATION OR DIARRHEA

Your partner should lie face down on the floor on a folded blanket, her arms at her sides, her forehead resting on a small stiff pillow or folded towel.

Head and Neck

Begin this sequence by kneeling above your partner's head, close enough so that you can comfortably reach the top of her head.

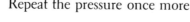

1 Place your right thumb on the point at the top center of the crown and place your left thumb on top of the right thumbnail. Give deep (20-pound) pressure for three seconds. Press in the direction of the spine. Pause.

2 Repeat the deep pressure in the direction of the spine. Pause.

3 Repeat the pressure once more.

Change your position and stand or kneel astride your partner with your weight on your lower legs.

4 Place your right thumb in the hollow at the base of the skull where the top of the neck joins the skull. Put your left thumb on top of the right. Give deep (20-pound) pressure for three seconds. Pause.

5 Repeat the pressure two more times.

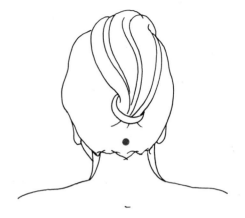

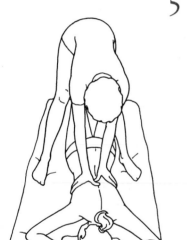

Bottom of the Spine

Move down so that you are straddling your partner's thighs and can easily reach the lower half of the spine. Run your thumb down the spine and feel the recesses between the vertebrae. You apply the pressure in these recesses, alternating thumbs, all the way from above the waistline to the bottom of the spine. Give pressure with your arms extended and the weight of your upper body transmitted down to and through your thumbs.

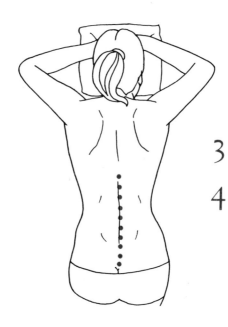

1 Place your right thumb in the recess four or five finger-widths above the waistline. Give moderate (15-pound) pressure for three seconds. Pause.

2 Place your left thumb in the next recessed point down the spine. Give moderate pressure for three seconds. Pause.

3 Continue down the spine to the tailbone, alternating thumbs in the recesses of the spine, giving moderate (15-pound) pressure at each point.

4 Repeat the above sequence (steps 1 to 3) two more times.

Right and Left Sides of the Spine

Without changing your position, place your left thumb immediately to the right side of the spine, four or five finger-widths above the waistline, and place your right thumb two finger-widths further to the right.

1 Give moderate (15-pound) pressure with both thumbs for three seconds. Pause.

2 Move both thumbs two finger-widths straight down alongside the spine. Repeat the pressure. Pause.

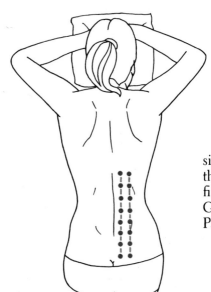

3 Continue down the right side of the spine at two finger-width intervals. Give moderate (15-pound) pressure for three seconds, pause, then continue, ending at a point midway down the buttock.

4 Repeat the above sequence (steps 1 to 3) two more times.

5 Now work on your partner's left side. Place your right thumb immediately to the left side of the spine, four or five finger-widths above the waistline. Place your left thumb two finger-widths further to the left on the same line. Give moderate (15-pound) pressure for three seconds. Pause.

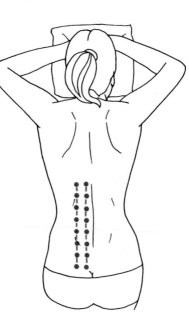

6 Move both thumbs two finger-widths straight down the left side of the spine and repeat the pressure.

7 Continue down the left side of the spine at two finger-width intervals. Give moderate (15-pound) pressure for three seconds at each point, pause, then continue, ending in the middle of the left buttock.

8 Repeat the above sequence (steps 5 to 7) two more times.

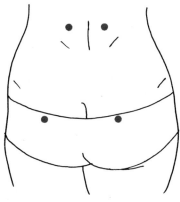

Hips

There are two points on each hip that receive shiatzu pressure. The first point is on the waistline, midway between the spine and the curve of the waist. The second point is on the buttock. First do the right side.

1 Kneel at your partner's right side. Place your left thumbtip on top of your right thumbtip on the point on the waistline. Give moderate (15-pound) pressure. Pause.

2 Repeat the pressure two more times. This is usually a tight point, so press until you feel it relax.

3 Move your hands down and place your thumbs side by side on a point just above the fleshiest part of the buttock in a direct line with the shoulder blades. Give moderate (15-pound) pressure for three seconds. Pause.

4 Repeat the pressure two more times.

5 Move over to your partner's left side and repeat the above sequence (steps 1 to 4) on the corresponding points on the left side.

Neck

Have your partner turn over and rest on her back. Kneel at the right side of her upper body, close enough so you can comfortably reach the neck without stretching your arms. The specific points in the illustration are only for general guidance. The idea is to cover the neck area thoroughly. Just cover the general area, starting beneath the jaw and working down to the base of the neck. Use the index and middle fingers of both hands, alternating your right and left hands.

1   Place the index and middle fingers of your right hand under the jaw beside the top of the windpipe. Give light (10-pound) pressure at the top of the line made by the windpipe and the neck muscle. Be careful not to press directly on the windpipe, but into the muscle. Hold for two seconds. Pause.

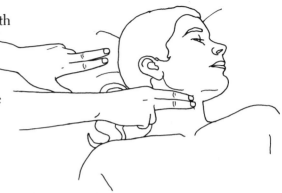

2   Place the index and middle fingers of your left hand just below the point you have just pressed with your right hand. Repeat the light pressure.

3   Continue to move straight down alongside the windpipe, alternating your hands to give light pressure, until you reach the base of the neck.

4   Bring your hands back up to the top of the neck underneath the jaw. Repeat the light (10-pound) pressures, alternating your hands, along a descending line to the base of the neck.

5   Continue the light (10-pound) pressures from the top of the neck to the base until you have covered the right side of the neck.

6   Move over to your partner's left side and repeat the sequence (steps 1 to 5) on the left side of the neck.

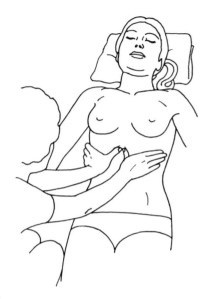

Abdomen

Kneel next to your partner's right hip so that you can easily reach the abdomen from the bottom of the rib cage to the tops of the legs. The points on the abdomen lie along five lines running from the bottom of the rib cage to the base of the trunk. Press corresponding points on both sides simultaneously.

1 Place both thumbs side by side just below the breastbone. Give moderate (15-pound) pressure for three seconds. Pause.

2 Move halfway down to the navel on the center line. Repeat the moderate pressure. Pause.

3 Continue down the center line at consistent intervals, giving moderate pressure for three seconds at each point, until you reach the groin.

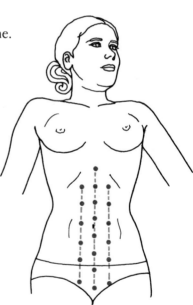

4 Separate your thumbs and place them at the waistline, four finger-widths to each side of the center line. Give moderate (15-pound) pressure simultaneously for three seconds. Pause.

5 Continue down the lines at two finger-width intervals. Give moderate pressure for three seconds at each pair of points, pause, then continue, ending at the groin.

6　Move your thumbs back to the waistline, four finger-widths further out toward the sides. Give moderate (15-pound) pressure for three seconds. Pause.

7　Continue down at two finger-width intervals, ending at the tops of the legs. Give moderate pressure at each point.

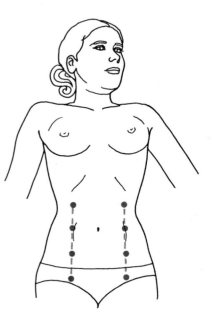

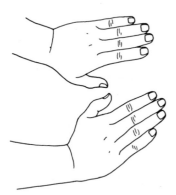

Kneel beside your partner's abdomen and place both hands on it, palms down. Give light (10-pound) and even pressure with both palms simultaneously, using your hands to cover the abdomen with gentle pressure. Pay particular attention to the lower part of the abdomen.

Final Exercises

Have your partner extend her arms out on the floor above her head. Grip her hands and pull gently, stretching her arms. At the same time she should inhale through her nose, filling her lungs to capacity, while stretching her legs and toes. Hold a moment, then release the tension on her hands while she exhales slowly through her mouth, relaxing her whole body. Repeat this exercise six times.

Chapter 12

Tennis Elbow

Shiatzu can speed your recovery from the disability and pain of tennis elbow. Tennis elbow or tendonitis of the elbow happens to people whose arm muscles become tight, usually from constant exertion. In this tightened condition, unnatural, or less than fluid, movement of the elbow can cause the tendons which connect the arm muscles to the elbow to compensate for the loss of muscle elasticity by stretching. This causes inflammation of the tendon at the joint. The attendant pain is a result of pressure from the tendon on the ulnar nerve, which is located at the inside rear point of the elbow. Shiatzu can help you with the immediate problem of the tendon inflammation.

In treating someone for tennis elbow, I give deep pressure to the shoulders and then throughout the affected arm. I give particular attention to the elbow joint. Shiatzu at or near the troubled joint is painful at first but the pain diminishes rather quickly. I recommend that shiatzu be given at least twice daily—in the morning and again at night before you go to bed. If you have the time, however, you should use shiatzu every three or four hours throughout the day. It will speed your recovery. After the whole sequence of exercises is completed, I always go back to the sensitive elbow points and give a few additional pressures. I also recommend that you refrain from playing for a few days until you have removed all of the soreness.

You can greatly minimize the risk of recurrence, or of being bothered by tennis elbow in the first place, by using shiatzu before and after each turn on the tennis court. It takes only a few minutes and puts the muscles of your shoulders and arms in a properly relaxed and elastic state.

I have also found that you can make shiatzu for tennis elbow particularly effective by soaking the affected area both before and after treatment. You can do this by placing your elbow under a faucet and running warm—not hot—water over the elbow, with strong pressure, for two or three minutes.

The shiatzu for tennis elbow exercises which follow are described in terms of an inflamed right elbow. If it is the left arm that is troubled, just reverse the instructions, i.e., right hand on left arm.

SELF-SHIATZU FOR TENNIS ELBOW

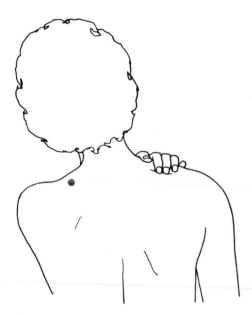

While the illustrations for this section presuppose that you are doing the sequences in the privacy of your home, they can be done anywhere, even while you are waiting for your turn on the court. They should be done while you are sitting on a chair or bench.

Shoulders

Find the point on top of your right shoulder with the index and middle fingers of your left hand. The point is halfway between the base of the neck and the edge of the shoulder. Probe slightly to the rear of the shoulder muscle with your fingers. When you are on the most tender spot you have found the point.

1 Give deep (20-pound) pressure for three seconds. Pause. Repeat the pressure two more times.

2 Locate the corresponding point on your left shoulder with the fingers of your right hand. Give deep pressure for three seconds. Repeat the pressure two more times.

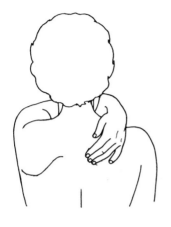

Upper Spine and Shoulder Blades

You will have to stretch to get to these points. Reach your left hand over your right shoulder as far down your back as you can. Your index finger should be just to the right of the spine.

1 Give deep (20-pound) pressure for three seconds with your index, middle and third fingers. Pause.

2 Move two finger-widths straight up the side of the spine and repeat the pressure. Pause.

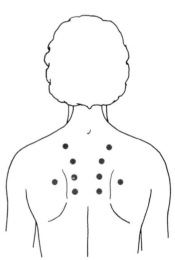

3 Continue up along the side of the spine at two finger-width intervals until you reach the shoulder line. Give deep pressure at each point for three seconds.

4 Place the index, middle and third fingers of your left hand in the center of the shoulder blade, inside the ridge of the shoulder blade. Give deep (20-pound) pressure for three seconds.

5 Repeat the sequence on the corresponding points on the left side. If your tennis elbow is too painful, skip this.

The balance of the exercises in this section are for a right-handed player. Simply use your right hand on your left arm if you are a left-handed player.

Armpit

Raise your right arm and place your left thumb deep in the armpit.

1   Give deep (20-pound) pressure for three seconds.

Outside of the Upper Arm

Place the index, middle and third fingers of your left hand on the center of the outside of the right arm, two finger-widths below the top of the shoulder. Wrap your thumb around the underside of the arm. The points run down the center of the outside of the upper arm from the shoulder to the elbow.

1   Give deep (20-pound) pressure for three seconds. Pause.

2   Move two finger-widths down the center line and repeat the pressure. Pause.

3   Continue down the center line at two finger-width intervals until you reach the elbow.

Outside of the Elbow

Bend your right arm at the elbow. Place your left index and middle fingers in the "ditch" between the two bones in the outer corner of the elbow.

1   Give deep (20-pound) pressure for three seconds. Pause.

2 Repeat the pressure two more times.

Outside of the Lower Arm

These points run from the outside of the elbow straight down to the center of the wrist.

1 Place your left thumb in the hollow on the outside of the right elbow, cradling your elbow in your fingers. Give deep (20-pound) pressure with your thumb for three seconds. Pause.

2 Move your thumb two finger-widths down the outside of the long muscle running down the forearm. Give deep pressure for three seconds. Pause.

3 Continue down this line at two finger-width intervals until you reach the wrist. The center of the back of the wrist is the last point.

Back of the Wrist

There are three points running like a bracelet along the back of the wrist in the hollows below the wrist bone. Press with your thumb.

1 Place your thumb on the first point below the base of the thumb. Give moderate (15-pound) pressure for three seconds. Pause.

2 Move your thumb over to the center of the wrist and repeat the pressure. Pause.

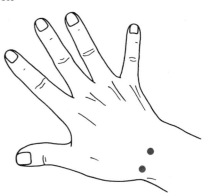

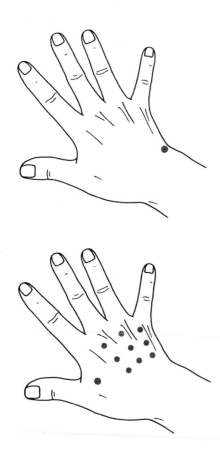

3 Move your thumb over to the point just below the wrist bone and repeat the pressure. Pause.

4 Repeat the sequence two more times.

Back of the Hand

Spread the fingers of your right hand. The points are located in the "ditches" between the tendons which run from your wrist to the first knuckles of each of your fingers.

1 Place your left thumb on the mound of muscle above the hollow at the base of the thumb where it joins the hand. Place your left index finger underneath your hand directly opposite your left thumb. Give deep (20-pound) pressure, squeezing with your thumb and index finger, for three seconds. Pause.

2 Repeat the pressure two more times.

3 Move your left thumb to the ditch between your index and middle fingers, midway between the wrist and the knuckle. Give moderate (15-pound) pressure for three seconds. Pause.

4 Moving down the ditch, repeat the pressure at two more points, ending between the knuckles.

5 Repeat the entire sequence in the ditches between the tendons leading to the middle and third fingers, then in the ditches between the third and little fingers.

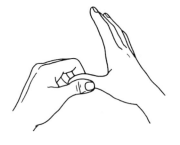

Fingers

Your thumb and each of your fingers should receive pressure at the top, bottom and sides of each of the individual bones—midway between the joints.

1 Grasp the front and back of the first joint of your right thumb between your left thumb and forefinger. Give moderate (15-pound) squeezing pressure for three seconds.

2 Move your left thumb up to the base of your right thumbnail. Place your left index finger directly opposite. Give moderate (15-pound) squeezing pressure for three seconds.

3 Grasp the sides of the first joint of your right thumb between your left thumb and forefinger. Give moderate (15-pound) pressure for three seconds. Pause.

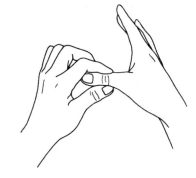

4 Move thumb and forefinger to the sides of the right thumbnail. Repeat the pressure.

5 Give pressure to each of your fingers in the same manner. Press the first and second joints of each finger, first on top and bottom, then along the sides. Then move on to the next finger.

Inside of the Upper Arm

The points on the inside of the upper arm lie along the top of the biceps muscle which runs down the center of the arm to the inside center of the elbow.

1 Place your left thumb at the top of the arm muscle. Wrap your fingers around the arm. Give deep (20-pound) pressure for two seconds. Pause.

2 Move two finger-widths down the center of the muscle and repeat the pressure. Pause.

3 Continue down the line at two finger-width intervals until you reach the inside center of the elbow.

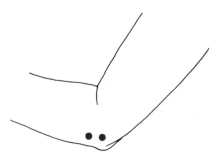

Inside of the Elbow

Bend your right arm at the elbow. Place your left thumb in the "ditch" between the two bones of the inside corner of the elbow. This is an extremely sensitive point, your "funny bone." When you press it, it should feel like an electric shock running from your elbow through your little finger.

1 Give deep (20-pound) pressure for two seconds. Pause.

2 Repeat the pressure two more times.

3 Move your thumb down an inch toward the wrist. Give deep (20-pound) pressure for two seconds. Pause.

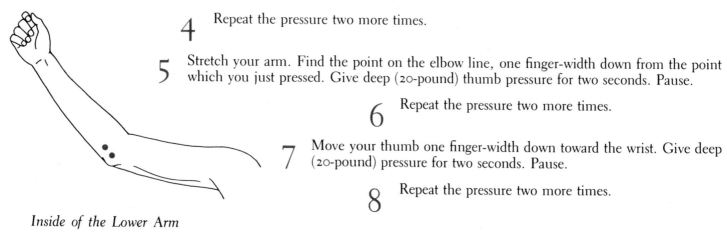

4 Repeat the pressure two more times.

5 Stretch your arm. Find the point on the elbow line, one finger-width down from the point which you just pressed. Give deep (20-pound) thumb pressure for two seconds. Pause.

6 Repeat the pressure two more times.

7 Move your thumb one finger-width down toward the wrist. Give deep (20-pound) pressure for two seconds. Pause.

8 Repeat the pressure two more times.

Inside of the Lower Arm

The points on the lower arm lie along a line which runs from the inside center of the elbow straight down the inside of the arm to the center of the wrist.

1 Place your left thumb on the inside center of the elbow. Wrap your fingers around the arm. Give deep (20-pound) pressure for two seconds. Pause.

2 Move two finger-widths down the line bisecting the inside of the forearm. Give deep pressure for two seconds. Pause.

3 Continue down this line at two finger-width intervals until you reach the wrist. The inside center of the wrist is the last point.

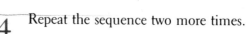

4 Repeat the sequence two more times.

Inside of the Wrist

There are three points along a horizontal line on the inside of the wrist.

1 Place your left thumb on your wrist, below the base of your thumb. Wrap your fingers around the back of your wrist. Give moderate (15-pound) pressure for three seconds. Pause.

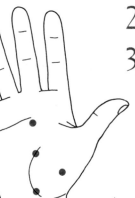

2 Move your thumb over to the center of the wrist and repeat the pressure. Pause.

3 Move your thumb over one more finger-width and repeat the pressure.

4 Repeat the sequence two more times.

Palm

There are four points on the palm. The first three lie along a line which runs from the heel of the hand to the base of the middle finger. The fourth point is at the center of the base of the thumb.

1 Place your left thumb in the center of the fleshy area at the base of the palm. Wrap your fingers around the back of your hand. Give deep (20-pound) pressure for three seconds. Pause.

2 Move your thumb down to the point in the center of the palm in a direct line with the first point. Repeat the pressure. Pause.

3 Move your thumb down to the fleshy area at the base of the middle finger and repeat the deep pressure. Pause.

4 Move your thumb to the point at the base of the thumb and repeat the pressure.

PARTNER-SHIATZU FOR TENNIS ELBOW

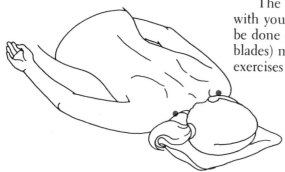

The instructions which follow assume that the exercises are being done at home, with your partner lying on the floor on a blanket. However, the sequences can readily be done elsewhere. The first three exercises (for the shoulders, upper spine and shoulder blades) may be done with your partner leaning against a wall. The balance of the exercises can be adjusted to a person sitting in a chair.

Shoulders

Have your partner lie face down. Kneel above her head, close enough so that you can reach the tops of her shoulders without stretching. The shoulder point is located three or four finger-widths out from the base of the neck. It is next to the knob of bone on the top of the shoulder and slightly to the rear.

1 Reach out your left arm and probe with your thumb until you find the point on the right shoulder. Place the bulb of your right thumb on top of your left thumbnail. Give deep (20-pound) pressure for three seconds. Pause.

2 Repeat the pressure two more times.

3 Reverse your thumbs and place your right thumb on the corresponding point on the left shoulder. Give deep (20-pound) pressure. Pause.

4 Repeat the pressure two more times.

Upper Spine

Stand astride your partner, facing her head, with your feet on a line with her hips. Bend down from your waist, flexing your knees, and place your left thumb immediately to the right of the spine, just below the big bulging vertebra at the base of the neck. Place your right thumb two finger-widths to the right on the same line.

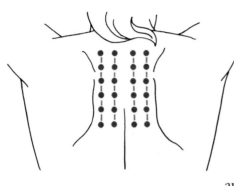

1 Give moderate (15-pound) pressure with both thumbs for three seconds. Pause.

2 Move both thumbs two finger-widths straight down the spine and repeat the pressure. Pause.

3 Continue down the side of the spine at two finger-width intervals until you are on a line with the middle of the shoulder blade.

4 Now place your right thumb on the shoulder line one finger-width to the left of the spine, place your left thumb two finger-widths further to the left, and repeat the sequence (steps 1 to 3) on the corresponding points on the left side of the spine.

Shoulder Blades

Place both your thumbs side by side in the center of the right shoulder blade, inside the edge of the shoulder blade.

1 Give moderate (15-pound) pressure for three seconds. Pause.

2 Repeat the pressure two more times.

3 Move both your thumbs to a point on the back of the shoulder, about three finger-widths above the armpit. Give moderate (15-pound) pressure with both thumbs for three seconds. Press upward toward the corner of the shoulder, against the bones of the shoulder joint. Pause.

4 Repeat the pressure two more times.

5 Repeat the sequence (steps 1 to 4) on the corresponding points on the left shoulder blade.

The sequences which follow assume that your partner is right-handed. The sequences should of course be applied to the left arm if she is a left-handed player.

Armpit

Have your partner turn over and rest on her back. Kneel at her right. Have her move her arm out from her body. Place your right thumb deep in your partner's armpit.

1 Give deep (20-pound) pressure for three seconds.

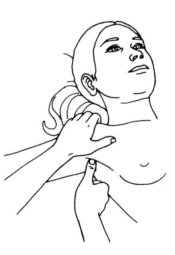

Outside of the Upper Arm

Place both your thumbs side by side on the center of the outside of the arm, two finger-widths below the top of the shoulder. Wrap your fingers around the arm.

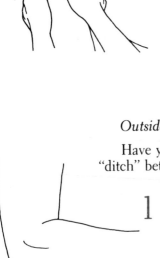

1 Give deep (20-pound) pressure with both thumbs for three seconds. Pause.

2 Move both thumbs two finger-widths down the center line toward the elbow and repeat the pressure. Pause.

3 Continue down the center line at two finger-width intervals until you reach the elbow.

Outside of the Elbow

Have your partner bend her right arm at the elbow. Place your thumb in the "ditch" between the two bones in the outer corner of the elbow.

1 Give deep (20-pound) pressure for three seconds. Pause.

2 Repeat the pressure two more times.

Outside of the Lower Arm

The points on the lower arm run on a line from the outside of the elbow straight down the center of the back of the forearm to the center of the wrist.

1 Place your thumbs side by side in the hollow on the outside of the elbow. Wrap your fingers around the arm.

2 Give deep (20-pound) pressure with both thumbs for three seconds. Pause.

3 Move two finger-widths down the outside of the long muscle running down the forearm. Give deep pressure for three seconds. Pause.

4 Continue down this line at two finger-width intervals until you reach the wrist. The center of the back of the wrist is the last point.

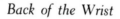

Back of the Wrist

There are three points on the back of the wrist. The first is at the right side of the wrist. The second is in the center. The third point is on the left side of the back of the wrist, below the base of the thumb. Hold your partner's wrist in one hand and give pressure with the thumb of the other.

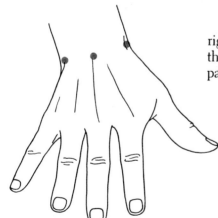

1 Place your thumb on the first point. Give moderate (15-pound) pressure for three seconds. Pause.

2 Move your thumb over to the center of the wrist and repeat the pressure. Pause.

3 Move your thumb over to the point below the base of the thumb and repeat the pressure. Pause.

4   Repeat the sequence two more times.

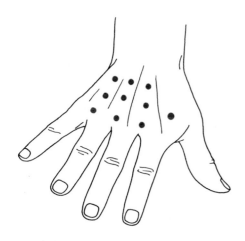

Back of the Hand

The points on the back of the hand are located in the "ditches" between the tendons which run from the wrist to the first knuckles of the fingers. Have your partner spread her fingers.

1   Place your thumb on the mound of muscle above the hollow at the base of the thumb where it joins the hand. Place your index finger underneath the hand, directly opposite your thumb.

2   Squeeze with deep (20-pound) pressure for three seconds. Pause.

3   Repeat the pressure two more times.

4   Move your thumb to the ditches between the tendons of the index and middle fingers, midway between the wrist and the knuckles. Give moderate (15-pound) pressure for three seconds. Pause.

5   Moving down the ditch, repeat the squeezing pressure at two more points, ending between the knuckles.

6   Repeat the entire sequence in the ditches between the tendons leading to the middle and third fingers, then in the ditches between the third and little fingers.

234   *Tennis Elbow*

Fingers

Give pressure to the thumb and each of the fingers at the top, bottom and sides of each of the individual bones, midway between the joints.

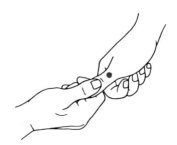

1 Grasp the front and back of the first joint of your partner's thumb between your thumb and forefinger. Give moderate (15-pound) squeezing pressure for two seconds. Pause.

2 Move up to the base of the thumbnail and repeat the pressure. Pause.

3 Move down and grasp the sides of her thumb between your fingers. Repeat the pressure. Pause.

4 Move to the sides of the thumbnail and repeat the pressure. Pause.

5 Give pressure to each of your partner's fingers in the same manner. Press the first and second joints of each finger, first on top and bottom, then along the sides. Then move on to the next finger.

Inside of the Upper Arm

Kneel a few feet away from your partner's midsection so that you can comfortably work on the upper arm. Have your partner extend her arm away from the side of her body, palm up. The points lie on a line which runs down the center of the upper arm muscle, from the armpit line to the inside center of the elbow.

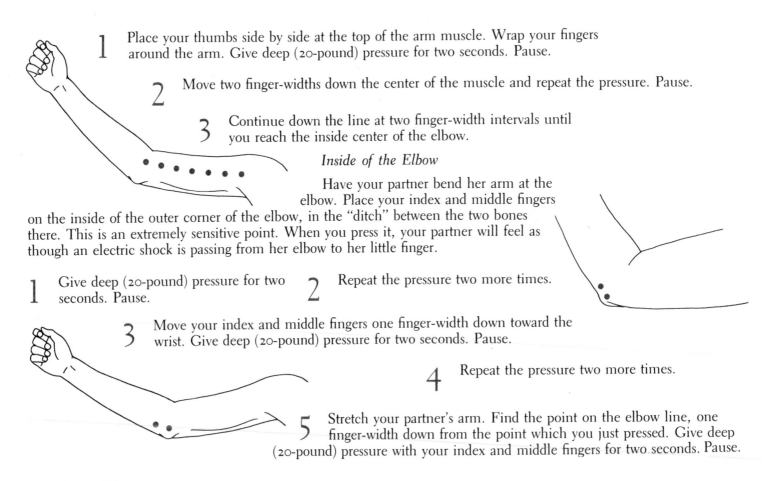

1   Place your thumbs side by side at the top of the arm muscle. Wrap your fingers around the arm. Give deep (20-pound) pressure for two seconds. Pause.

2   Move two finger-widths down the center of the muscle and repeat the pressure. Pause.

3   Continue down the line at two finger-width intervals until you reach the inside center of the elbow.

Inside of the Elbow

Have your partner bend her arm at the elbow. Place your index and middle fingers on the inside of the outer corner of the elbow, in the "ditch" between the two bones there. This is an extremely sensitive point. When you press it, your partner will feel as though an electric shock is passing from her elbow to her little finger.

1   Give deep (20-pound) pressure for two seconds. Pause.

2   Repeat the pressure two more times.

3   Move your index and middle fingers one finger-width down toward the wrist. Give deep (20-pound) pressure for two seconds. Pause.

4   Repeat the pressure two more times.

5   Stretch your partner's arm. Find the point on the elbow line, one finger-width down from the point which you just pressed. Give deep (20-pound) pressure with your index and middle fingers for two seconds. Pause.

236   *Tennis Elbow*

6 Repeat the pressure two more times.

7 Move your index and middle fingers one finger-width down toward the wrist. Give deep (20-pound) pressure for two seconds. Pause.

8 Repeat the pressure two more times.

Inside of the Lower Arm

The points on the lower arm lie along a line which runs from the inside center of the elbow straight down the inside of the arm to the center of the wrist.

1 Place your thumbs side by side on the inside center of the elbow. Wrap your fingers lightly around the joint. Give deep (20-pound) pressure for two seconds. Pause.

2 Move two finger-widths down the line bisecting the inside of the forearm. Give deep pressure for two seconds. Pause.

3 Continue down this line at two finger-width intervals until you reach the wrist. The inside center of the wrist is the last point.

4 Repeat the sequence two more times.

Inside of the Wrist

There are three points along a horizontal line on the inside of the wrist.

1 Place your thumb on your partner's wrist, below the base of her thumb. Hold her hand in your other hand.

2 Give moderate (15-pound) pressure for three seconds. Pause.

3 Move your thumb over to the center of the wrist and repeat the pressure. Pause.

4 Move your thumb over one more finger-width and repeat the pressure.

5 Repeat the sequence two more times.

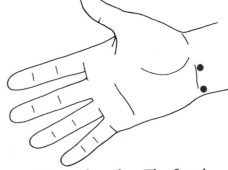

Palm

There are four points on the palm. The first three lie along a line which runs from the heel of the hand to the base of the middle finger. The fourth point is at the center of the base of the thumb.

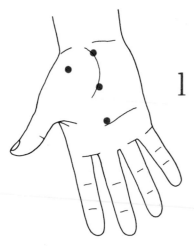

1 Place both your thumbs side by side in the center of the fleshy area at the base of the palm. Give deep (20-pound) pressure with both thumbs for three seconds. Pause.

2 Move down to the point in the center of the palm in a direct line with the first point. Repeat the pressure. Pause.

3 Move your thumbs down to the fleshy area at the base of the middle finger and repeat the deep pressure. Pause.

4 Move your thumbs to the point at the base of the thumb and repeat the pressure.

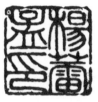

Afterword

I want to tell you more about shiatzu,
but space has run out. However, you now have a
thorough explanation of its fundamentals.
Follow the programs faithfully and consistently,
and you will feel better, look younger
and have more vigor.

Goseiko o inorimasu! Good luck and success!

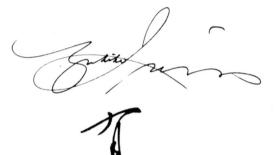

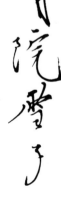

About the Author

Yukiko Irwin, a sixth-generation direct descendant of Benjamin Franklin, has practiced shiatzu for twenty-five years, ten of them in New York City on referrals from physicians. She is a graduate of the Nippon Shiatzu School in Tokyo, Tokyo Woman's Christian College, and Indiana University. She is also a member of the Japanese Medical Society of New York. Her patients include many of the public figures of our time, and she has served as resident therapist of a major ballet company.